BREECH BIRTH

Benna Waites

Illustrations by Anthony Craib

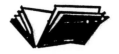

FREE ASSOCIATION BOOKS / LONDON / NEW YORK

First published in Great Britain in 2003 by
FREE ASSOCIATION BOOKS
57 Warren Street
London W1T 5NR

www.fabooks.com

A catalogue record for this book is available from the British Library

ISBN 1 85343 563 5

10   9   8   7   6   5   4   3   2   1

Produced for Free Association Books by
Chase Publishing Services, Fortescue, Sidmouth EX10 9QG
Printed and bound by CPI Antony Rowe, Eastbourne

For Jasper, my own breech baby, who started it all

Contents

List of Tables

List of Figures

Foreword

Wendy Savage

This is an excellent book which I would recommend not only for women who find themselves with a breech presentation near the end of pregnancy (term), but also to all medical students, qualified and student midwives, consultants and trainees in obstetrics.

The vast majority of babies which present by the breech at term – this happens to about 1 in 30 women – are perfectly normal and healthy and the mechanism of breech delivery is such that babies can safely be born bottom first as long as the doctor or midwife understands this and has been trained in how to assist at the birth. Basically this means allowing the uterine contractions to push the baby down the birth canal and interfering as little as possible. Although no randomised trials have been conducted of the best position to give birth to a baby presenting by the breech it seems likely that the upright or kneeling position is physiologically and anatomically better than the modern lithotomy position (where the woman lies on her back with her legs supported in stirrups). The latter is unfortunately the way that most doctors today have been taught how to deliver babies presenting by the breech although with the increasing use of caesarean section for delivery in the last decade in the UK, many have little if any training in how to perform a breech delivery.

Breech presentation has always raised some anxieties in both women and their doctors because before the days of prenatal screening and routine ultrasound examinations in the second trimester of pregnancy babies with serious congenital abnormalities such as anencephaly with or without spina bifida (a condition where the brain does not develop fully or the spine does not fuse so exposing nerve tissue) and hydrocephaly (water on the brain) were not always identified. Today these conditions would in a developed country like the UK be detected ante-natally and the woman offered a termination of pregnancy with anencephaly which is incompatible with survival, or an elective caesarean section with hydrocephaly, when the head is large so that drainage of the fluid can be done when the baby is born in the hope that the brain has not been damaged by the increased pressure.

Although before ultrasound obstetricians used X-rays if hydrocephaly was suspected, lesser degrees might not be detected before birth and it is the "folk memory", which I think is responsible for the fear that the head will get stuck once the body of the baby has been delivered. At term the width of the baby's hips is similar to that of the greatest width of the head (the bi-parietal diameter or BPD) so if the bottom of the baby has gone through the pelvis so should the head. However, I have heard trainees telling women that this may happen which is a frightening thought for any woman discussing the options available to her. Personally I have only once experienced this complication and this was in Kenya where a woman came in having had no ante-natal care and had already pushed the body of the baby out on her way to hospital and it is possible that her relatives may have pulled on the body and extended the head. I did an emergency symphysiotomy and delivered the baby, as there was still a fetal heart. No post-mortem was done and no measurements of the head were possible in the neonatal unit where the baby survived for a few hours. When I have asked practising obstetricians about their experience since ultrasound scanning (USS) and prenatal screening became routine I have yet to find one who has been in this situation.

There is one other problem, which rarely occurs – that of the nuchal arm. In this case (which may well be encouraged by pulling on the trunk of the baby early in the process of birth), an arm may be extended behind the baby's neck thus making it difficult for the head to come down into the pelvis. I have never had this experience in 35 years of obstetric practice but I have watched a video where Ina May Gaskin dealt with this calmly and competently by running her finger along the baby's arm and sweeping the arm down over the cheek so that the head could descend. Ina May Gaskin is the leading co-author of *Spiritual Midwifery* based on the experience of the self-taught midwives at the Farm in Tennessee. These midwives have achieved excellent results[1] and most of the babies born on the Farm were born at home although they had a house set up for births such as twins or breech deliveries where, still in a homely setting, there was more space and a little more equipment.

The secret of a successful breech delivery is to keep one's hand off the baby and let nature take its course. The teaching was to "sit on your hands". The woman needs to understand that after pushing the body down she must then let the head come down slowly as pressure changes if the head leaves the constricted bony pelvic canal and enters the open air too rapidly which may lead to bleeding inside the baby's skull. This is a very rare complication and probably more likely if the baby is premature. I have never had a woman who, having had it explained to her that we do not want the baby's head to come out like "a cork out of a bottle", has not been able to stop pushing when asked to do so. The reason that many obstetricians have insisted on an epidural and controlling the descent of the head by applying forceps is to prevent sudden pressure changes but unfortunately this is not usually explained to the woman, who is quite capable of controlling this herself.

The second important part in training doctors and midwives to assist in delivering the breech vaginally is to look at the clock when the baby's head enters the pelvis. At this point the cord is compressed and so little oxygen is going to the baby. Babies are designed to be born and are able to survive much longer than adults without oxygen to the brain; probably five rather than two minutes. They do this by using anaerobic respiration. However, the stimulus to the brain of the carbon dioxide, which is accumulating, does make the baby attempt to breathe as the head descends and the body hangs down. This makes inexperienced birth attendants anxious. The time seems endless as the body comes down slowly but if you look at the clock you see that only 10 or 20 seconds have passed. This reassurance stops the doctor or midwife from trying to deliver the baby faster thus risking extension of the head

1. Durand, A.M. (1992) The safety of home birth: the Farm study. *American Journal of Public Health* 82: 450–2.

and converting a normal and successful mechanism into one where it becomes more difficult to deliver the baby, force is used and the catalogue of complications which are listed in the textbooks become more likely.

This book clearly explains the literature and the options available to women who find that the baby is "upside-down" near term. As doctors have become less confident about breech delivery the possibility of turning the baby round, external cephalic version, has become more popular again and the pros and cons of this manoeuvre are explained in the text.

The Midirs leaflet about breech birth published about six years ago suggested at that time that because of the uncertainty about the best way to deliver a baby presenting by the breech, the woman should decide after having had the options explained, how she wanted to give birth. Sadly I think there are very few women who get a positive view of the options and an example of the importance of the attitude of the obstetrician can be taken from my own hospital, the Royal London. Two thirds of women booked under my care who had a breech presentation delivered vaginally, half of those under the care of the colleague with whom I worked most closely and one third of the other three consultants. Overall about half of women booked at the London had a vaginal breech delivery, yet our two closest hospitals had much lower rates of vaginal breech delivery.

In 2000 the long awaited term breech randomised controlled trial was published in the *Lancet*[2] and commentators have considered that this gave women the best information about the risks of vaginal breech delivery compared with elective caesarean section (CS) and that all women should be offered an elective CS.[3] However, many of us who considered that with good selection and properly trained staff vaginal breech delivery was a safe option for women, and had rates of CS less than 50% had not entered their women into the trial as this would have been unethical. Only those who were genuinely unsure could subject at least 50% of women to an elective CS based on random allocation to one group or another. This means that those who were confident and practising vaginal breech delivery on a regular basis were unlikely to have taken part in the trial. This was terminated early because of concerns about the difference in perinatal mortality but a careful analysis of these deaths does make one question this decision and the conclusions reached. Roosmalen and Rosendaal, two Dutch obstetricians, writing in September 2002[4] do not accept the conclusion that all women should be encouraged to have a CS and point out that the well documented increased morbidity and mortality following CS were unlikely to be picked up in the short follow-up period of the study. Another criticism is the small number of cases entered by some centres in this multi-centre trial, which does not suggest that these were places where vaginal breech delivery

2. Hannah, M.E., et al. (2000) Planned caesarean versus planned vaginal birth for breech presentation at term: a randomised multicentre trial. *Lancet* 356: 1375–83.
3. Lumley, J. (2000) Any room left for disagreement about assisting breech births at term? *Lancet* 356: 1368–9; Shennan, A. and Bewley, S. (2001) How to manage term breech deliveries. Avoid vaginal breech deliveries but offer external cephalic version. *British Medical Journal* 323: 244–5.
4. Van Roosmalen, J. and Rosendaal, F. (2002) There is still room for disagreement about vaginal delivery of breech infants at term. *British Journal of Obstetrics and Gynaecology* 109: 967–9.

was routinely undertaken, yet experience, as explained above, is a crucial factor in achieving good outcomes. In addition there was much less difference between the outcomes in developing countries than in the developed ones, again suggesting that experience in breech delivery was an important factor.

In Scandinavia where large studies of breech births delivered vaginally have been published it seems unlikely that the policy of encouraging vaginal breech births for women who want them will change, despite this trial. Sadly many hospitals in the UK have stopped offering women the choice of vaginal breech delivery on the basis of the Hannah study so women's choice is further restricted.

This book will help you to make up your own mind about how you want to give birth to your "upside-down" baby and I hope you succeed in delivering vaginally like millions of women have done over the years.

Wendy Savage
20 April 2003

Acknowledgements

I would like to thank the following:

Donald Gibb who, in the first place, took me on as his patient and so skilfully helped me to give birth to my own breech baby, for which I shall be eternally grateful. His enthusiasm and support throughout the process of the book have been invaluable, from the genesis of the idea, to being interviewed, to his constructive feedback on the manuscript.

All the women who talked to me or wrote to me with their own experiences of breech. Reading about their experiences showed me that so many of them felt the same information gap as I had done and helped convince me that the book really would be worthwhile even if it helped just a few women in a similar situation. The book is far richer for their contribution. Also a big thank you to the women who allowed me to use their amazing birth photographs. As is the convention in such cases, the real names of these mothers and their babies have been changed for the purpose of confidentiality.

All the professionals who gave up their time to be interviewed for the book and share their own experiences of and opinions about breech. Their comments put flesh on the dry bones of so many of the concepts explored in the book.

Annie Francis, mother, midwife and ex-neighbour whose encouragement when I was pregnant and feedback and enthusiasm about the manuscript were inspiring.

Wendy Savage for detailed feedback on the manuscript and willingness to write a foreword.

The librarians at the Royal College of Obstetricians and Gynaecologists and at Queen Mary's University Hospital, for an efficient and friendly service.

My publisher, Trevor Brown, who, in a sea of dismissiveness, seemed genuinely excited by my proposal and seemed also to understand that it would take as long as it took and never hassled me.

My friends for continuing to be interested and excited about the book even as the years rolled by, Marion for childcare and help with references, my mother for believing in me, using her editorial eye on the entire manuscript and, along with Gran, handing down a tradition of good birth.

Above all, Anthony for drawings, detailed feedback as first reader, unwavering faith in me and my ability to get this book out of me, sharing my passion for the subject of breech and tolerating the inevitable impact writing a book like this has had upon our lives.

I also formally acknowledge the kind permission to reproduce the following illustrations:

Figure 2.1, reproduced with kind permission from Oxford University Press.

Figure 4.1, reproduced with kind permission from Westgren, M., Edvall, H., Nordstrom, L., Svalenius, E. and Ranstam, J. and *British Journal of Obstetrics and Gynaecology*.

Table 5.3, reproduced with kind permission from Elsevier Science.

Table 6.1, reproduced with kind permission from Hellstrom et al. and *Acta Obstetrica et Gynecologia Scandinavica.*

Table 6.2, reproduced with kind permission from Newbold, R.B. et al. and *American Journal of Obstetrics and Gynecology.*

Figure 7.1, reproduced with kind permission from Cardini, F., Basevi, V., Valentinie, A. and Martellato, A. and *American Journal of Chinese Medicine.*

Table 8.1, reproduced with kind permission from Elsevier Science.

Table 12.1, reproduced with kind permission from Free Association Books.

How to Use this Book

This booked is aimed at the heterogeneous audience of mothers and fathers of breech babies, midwives, medical students, obstetricians, ante-natal class teachers, alternative therapists and anyone with an interest in learning more about breech babies. This diversity has at times made it difficult to judge the level at which to present material and the amount of prior knowledge to assume. I have erred on the side of caution, trying to minimise assumptions about prior knowledge and trying to make language as accessible as possible. However, I have not avoided the inclusion of material that is at times complex and if there are times when you feel you are losing the plot somewhat, I apologise. As my primary purpose in writing the book was to render the vast amount of material available on breech comprehensible for parents who may, like me, find themselves late on in pregnancy with a breech baby and needing to consider their options in a hurry, I hope that non-medical readers do not feel too confused or overwhelmed too often.

All users of this book are likely at some points to feel that chunks of it are not relevant to them and I would urge a selective approach – fully utilising skim reading skills where necessary. I have deliberately provided fairly detailed introductions and summary sections at the beginning and ends of each chapter to help you to work out which bits are most relevant and useful to you. Frequent subheadings should help you to find your way through each chapter more easily.

I have attempted to be as thorough as I can be in my review of the research evidence on breech. I have also tried to present the research as critically as possible, helping you to become aware of what we can and cannot conclude from the available evidence. Alongside conclusions from research I have also presented the opinions of a range of midwife and obstetrician interviewees detailed at the beginning of this book. I have always aimed to make clear what is based on research, and what on opinion and hope that this combination of information sources does not cause any confusion. One of my concerns about the breech debate is that people often present opinion as fact, so I have endeavoured to avoid falling into the same trap myself.

If you are carrying twins, one or both of whom are breech, there may be aspects of this book which are relevant to you. However, to do justice to the immense subject of carrying and giving birth to twins, an entire book of its own is needed. I have not therefore attempted to deal with the subject of breech birth in twins directly. If your baby is lying transverse (i.e., across your uterus), some of parts one and two of this book are relevant to you. Transverse lie is not often mentioned directly because of lack of research on the topic, but much of the material in these early sections of the book is applicable to babies lying in a transverse position. Babies who stay in a transverse position cannot be born vaginally (though they may turn or be turned in labour) so subsequent sections are less relevant.

Apart from the introduction, the rest of the book has been referenced, with a number in brackets indicating the source of the statement made or the evidence upon which it is based. These sources are mainly journal articles and books but also include "personal communication" – obstetricians, midwives and others who have been kind enough to be interviewed for the book. The numbers are there for you to identify sources and follow up research where you wish to. The references include journal titles in full, rather than in abbreviated form, to facilitate research by the obstetrically uninitiated. However, it is fully anticipated that many of you, particularly lay readers, may have no wish to trace source material. In such cases, please ignore the numbers as best you can.

In spite of my best efforts, I am confident of countless imperfections throughout this book. If there is sufficient interest, there is a possibility of a subsequent edition to ensure the book remains up to date. In the light of this, any comments, criticisms, opinions, experiences that you would care to share with me would be greatly appreciated and can be sent to me via the publisher.

A Note on Language

To make this book as accessible as possible to my main target audience of parents I have tried to avoid the use of jargon. If this reads oddly to the professional reader, I apologise. It seemed important not to obscure what is at times already a fairly complex text with inaccessible language. Examples of this include an avoidance of the use of the term gestation (meaning pregnancy) and replacement of the terms cephalic or vertex with head down. The only exception to this is when the alternative is very clumsy or cumbersome. Although I have broadly tried to avoid the use of the terms parity (the number of pregnancies the woman has had), nulliparous/nulliparae (used to describe a woman in her first pregnancy) and multiparous/multiparae (a woman with one or more previous pregnancies), there are times when their inclusion enables the text to flow better. When used these terms have normally been explained immediately afterwards. Other examples of terms whose meanings may not be immediately apparent are mortality (death) and morbidity (complications or disease). Perinatal mortality refers to death around the time of birth (sometimes also called intrapartum death) and neonatal mortality refers to death within the first 28 days after birth.

If you are ever struggling to understand a word or concept, most pregnancy books include glossaries with a list of vocabulary used in pregnancy, or alternatively ask your midwife or doctor.

I have deliberately tried to avoid the use of the term fetus. Medical literature appears to use the term fetus up to the point of birth, at which point the terms infant or baby are used. My baby felt like a baby long before it was born and I have used the term baby throughout. I do not believe this will cause confusion as context normally clarifies whether the baby is born or unborn. I have used the term "it" rather than "he" or "she" to refer to your baby.

Finally a distinction is made throughout the book between vaginal birth and vaginal delivery. For reasons which should become clear, many people would argue that there is a fundamental difference between breech birth, in which the baby is born primarily through the efforts of mother and baby, and breech delivery in which the baby is delivered by a medical team, often with the use of forceps, an epidural and the lithotomy position.

Biographies of Interviewees

A number of professionals from the world of obstetrics and midwifery kindly agreed to be interviewed for the book, and their comments appear throughout. To give you some idea of who they are and from what context they approach the subject of breech, here are some brief details on their backgrounds and current situations.

Alice Coyle SRN, SCM, AIST, BSc (Hons): Alice has been a midwife since 1980, after previously qualifying as a nurse. She worked in the NHS for five years, during which time she gave birth to her two children, Jack and Kate. Jack was breech and delivered by emergency caesarean section at 30 weeks due to placenta abruptio (separated placenta). Subsequently she was found to have a bicornuate uterus (see Chapter 2) and a flattened sacrum (see Chapter 9) and was consequently persuaded to have an elective caesarean section for Kate's birth. She has been an independent midwife in Birth Rites, a busy South London Independent Midwifery Practice, where she has developed a particular interest in home birth, breech birth, vaginal birth after caesarean, natural twin birth and the little known/offered option of "caesarean after commencement of labour" as a substitute for elective caesarean section (see Chapters 11 and 12). She lectures both at home and abroad and assisted in establishing the first aquanatal classes in Britain. She has just completed a degree in anthropology which gave her fascinating insights into many aspects of the birthing process.

Mary Cronk RGN, RM, ABM, NCDN, MBE: Mary Cronk practised for many years as a district midwife and as an NHS community midwife. Since 1990 she has been an independent midwife based in Chichester. She has a particular interest in and experience of caring for women whose babies present by the breech and has lectured and written articles on the subject. In 1998 she was awarded an MBE for services to midwifery.

Jane Evans SRN, SCM: Jane Evans is an independent midwife with an interest in and many years of experience of breech birth, including breech birth at home.

Caroline Flint SRN, SCM, ADM: Caroline Flint has been a midwife for 26 years. She is the Director of the Birth Centre in Tooting, south west London and she runs a large independent midwifery practice which serves women all over London. Her passion is that women should have choice at all times during pregnancy, labour and post-natally. Her practice is very experienced in home births, water births, gentle births and births in a Birth Centre. She has written five books and over 300 articles and she lectures internationally.

Donald Gibb MD, MRCP, FRCOG, ME, WI: Donald Gibb is currently an Independent Consultant Obstetrician, working at the St John and St Elizabeth Hospital and the Portland Hospital in London. Prior to this he worked as an NHS consultant at King's College Hospital in London where he worked closely with both NHS and independent midwives who helped shape his current approach. This, along with exposure to "real obstetrics" in Singapore and Africa early in his career have left him critical of much modern obstetric practice. He left the NHS to work privately as he felt the NHS has difficulty delivering the level of personal care necessary for pregnant women. He remains positive and motivated about vaginal breech birth, in spite of the views and practices of many of his colleagues.

Yehudi Gordon MB, BCh, FRCOG, FCOG (SA): Yehudi Gordon is a Consultant Obstetrician working at the Birth Unit at the Hospital of St John and St Elizabeth in London. He was a founder member of the active birth movement and was one of the pioneers of active and water birth in the United Kingdom. He co-founded the Birth Unit where he now works which is dedicated to providing integrated healthcare for mothers and babies, including the use of conventional and complimentary medicine.

Michel Odent MD: Michel Odent is an obstetrician who spent the early part of his career in Pithiviers Hospital in France. With six midwives, he was responsible for around 1000 births per year. He was renowned for introducing the concept of home-like birthing rooms, the use of water in labour and childbirth and for low rates of intervention. He has attended approximately 300 breech births, two of which were at home. He has authored approximately 50 scientific papers and 10 books. He is now retired from clinical practice but continues to pursue research interests.

Wendy Savage MSc (Hons), DSc, FRCOG: Wendy Savage is an obstetrician now retired from clinical practice. She qualified from Cambridge and the London Hospital Medical School in 1960 and obtained her obstetric qualification in 1971 after spending time in Nigeria, Kenya and America. She became a senior lecturer and consultant at the London Hospital Medical College in 1977. In 1985 she was suspended on charges of incompetence which were later deemed groundless. She published her own account of these charges, two of which related to the management of vaginal breech labour, and the subsequent investigation, in her book *A Savage Enquiry.* In the same year she was elected a Fellow of the Royal College of Obstetricians and Gynaecologists and in 1986 she was reinstated as Honorary Consultant at the Royal London Hospital, where she stayed until her retirement in 2000. She became Honorary Visiting Professor at Middlesex University in 1991. She has been elected to various Committees and bodies through the 1990s to date including the General Medical Council, and has been on the Standards Professional Conduct and Professional Performance Committees. She was on the British Medical Association Council from 2000 to 2002. She has been the author or co-author of several books and papers. She has four children and four grandchildren and lives in London.

Guy Thorpe-Beeston MA, MD, FRCOG: Guy Thorpe-Beeston is a consultant obstetrician at the Chelsea and Westminster Hospital in London. He trained at Cambridge University and Guy's Hospital. His research has been into fetal medicine and he wrote a paper on breech while at St Mary's Hospital. He has maintained an interest in breech since then.

Introduction

There are many reasons for my writing this book, and I hope at least some of them correspond to your reasons for reading it.

In the last four weeks of my pregnancy with my first child, I was told that my baby was breech and that he was likely to stay that way. I was desperate for information about breech birth and started scanning the shelves of pregnancy sections in book shops and studying index pages of any pregnancy book I could lay my hands on. I was shocked by how little information there was available. There was no book devoted to the subject and every general pregnancy and birth book I found felt woefully brief in its approach to the subject. Look up breech in the index of any general text on pregnancy and birth and you will be referred to no more than a handful of page numbers spread throughout the book, often with a short paragraph that leaves you with more questions than answers. This was not enough. I wanted to know how every aspect of my pregnancy and birth planning was affected by my baby being breech. There is also the problem that the experience you have out there in your local hospital often does not correspond to what the book leads you to expect. It is all very well seeing diagrams of a vaginal breech birth in a semi-supported squat position (311), or reading about how you should be offered external cephalic version (see Chapter 5) to help your baby to turn (312), but generally there is little information given about what you can do if your consultant tells you to have a caesarean or says he doesn't do external cephalic version.

When I came to put forward my proposal for the book to publishers, I frequently received the response that the subject was too specialist for them. While this may well be the case if your job is to think about profits, if you are a pregnant woman with a breech baby it is your whole experience, not just a small part of it. The lack of a book on the subject seemed to heighten the sense of isolation that can already be so acute on finding out your baby is breech. Breech babies are sufficiently rare (approximately 3% of births) that you may not meet anyone else with one during your pregnancy. The sudden catapulting to "high risk" status from what will probably have been a perfectly normal pregnancy is an anxiety inducing and lonely business. Suddenly ante-natal classes, designed amongst other things to bring people together on the grounds of similar experience, can feel filled with people who have no inkling of what you are going through. I hope that by quoting directly from the women who have been kind enough to talk or write to me for this book, you may experience a little of the companionship that is lacking from most people's ante-natal breech experience.

A good chunk of this book is devoted to relatively uncontroversial information about the causes of breech and the various techniques for encouraging breech babies to turn. However, there is much of it that focuses on research on vaginal and caesarean breech birth. My reason for presenting so much information on the options for breech birth is quite simply that many obstetricians don't seem to be doing it. Scare stories and doom laden advice are relatively easy to access; balanced, objective, research based evidence and opinion are not. My disappointment with so many of the obstetric profession (with some notable and worthy exceptions) was another key reason for writing this book. Being kind, one might suggest that the lack of time National Health Service (NHS) consultants have available to them prevents the kind of discussion required when your baby is diagnosed as breech. Busy ante-natal clinics are not conducive to in depth discussions of the pros and cons of different birth options and how these are affected by a particular consultant's opinion and past experience. However, I believe the problem runs much deeper than this.

"Caesarean is best for baby" is a statement, generally presented as a fact, which often confronts the woman with a breech baby. This is far from fully justified by the evidence (see Chapter 8). Is it simply that "obstetricians are less scientific-minded than other medical specialists" as one obstetrician has suggested (268)? I had, naively perhaps, always believed medicine to be an evidence based profession. As a clinical psychologist working in the NHS I was aware of the increasing drive towards evidence based practice and audit. I assumed that practice was informed by research, and updated according to the latest findings. Indeed, so ready was I to trust the medical profession's expertise that I had rather shunned the idea of a birth plan early in my pregnancy as it seemed a rather arrogant way to approach an experience I had never had before and that obstetricians had witnessed hundreds of times. Surely, I assumed, I could trust them to take care of my baby's and my own best interests with an intelligent, evidence based approach?

As I hope will be clear from reading Chapter 8, there are few certainties when it comes to weighing up the options for breech birth. Even with the Canadian multi-centre international breech trial, published in 2000, paraded by some as delivering "the answer" to the breech conundrum (the answer apparently being to routinely offer caesarean section for breech), there is sufficient criticism of the study (see Chapter 8) to leave many feeling that the answer still eludes us. Overall the body of research we have often produces mutually conflicting data, and conclusions often state that studies of sufficient size and with good enough design have not yet been carried out. The active, spontaneous approach to vaginal breech birth, described in more detail in Chapter 10 and espoused by some as the only safe way to conduct a vaginal breech birth is yet to be properly evaluated. Uncertainty should therefore be the uncomfortable though realistic norm in cases of breech. As the late Peter Huntingford, an obstetrician notable for his eloquent criticism of his profession, has written:

For most doctors, the most truthful response they could give in many cases would be: ....This is the situation as I see it: we could do this or that, but I am not really sure which is best. Under these circumstances, what would you prefer me to do? (328)

However, such uncertainty does not sit easily with a profession used to giving advice and it is rare to find a consultant obstetrician willing to have this kind of conversation. It is far more likely that you will be instantly offered a management plan based on your new found "high risk" status, and that this plan will be presented as a set of rules from which it would be irresponsible to deviate.

Interestingly, breech was not always perceived as a dangerous or alarming occurrence. Wendy Savage told me an anecdote about an obstetrician in the 1930s in Chicago who managed his patients by turning all his head down presentations to breech prior to delivery, presumably because he found it easier that way (286). There appears to have been a growing "folk anxiety" (286) about breech which permeates large tracts of the general population as well as the midwifery and obstetric professions, and it is worth briefly exploring why it has taken hold so strongly.

One reason is that a higher percentage of breech babies are born with congenital abnormalities (malformations present at birth), though bear in mind that the vast majority are normal. For a while it may have been assumed that some of these problems were the result of a traumatic birth and therefore preventable with a caesarean. Only now that many studies comparing vaginal and caesarean births are starting to show little difference in outcomes for babies are people starting to question whether complications have been wrongly blamed on vaginal breech birth. There may be something about some abnormalities which make the baby more likely to lie in a breech position during pregnancy (see Chapter 2). If these abnormalities are not identified prior to birth, vaginal breech birth may have acquired a bad name for problems that were never in fact caused by it.

Another problem associated with breech is prematurity. More premature babies are breech simply because they haven't yet had a chance to settle into a head down position. Premature babies are more likely to have problems at birth. Again though, this is not the responsibility of a vaginal breech labour. It is true that premature babies have bigger heads in relation to the rest of their bodies which may require a premature breech labour to be more carefully managed and may increase the argument for caesarean in such cases (see Chapter 7), though this too is controversial. However, this should not affect the management of term breech babies whose heads and bottoms have comparable diameters (286).

Another significant cause of folk anxiety about breech birth is mismanagement stemming from anxiety and inexperience. The dangers of this leading to pulling on the baby and the damage that this can cause is documented in Chapter 9.

There are other reasons for caesareans being performed more readily for breech which relate to the general increase in caesarean section across the developed world. Medico-legal concerns, convenience (both women's and obstetricians') and technological intervention have all served to increase the caesarean rate beyond a level which produces any corresponding improvement in infant outcomes. The authors of one study caution:

> The present medico-legal climate can penalize poor neonatal outcome, regardless of cause, but rarely penalizes unnecessary surgery. This could stimulate doctors to practise defensive medicine leading to increased rates of caesarean section. (261)

I would not want to fail to accord caesarean section the respect that its considered use deserves. Indeed, reviewing the history of obstetric intervention in birth, it could perhaps be claimed that caesarean section is among the greatest obstetric achievements. With ultrasound it is now possible to detect breech babies who may have problems being born vaginally such as those with minor degrees of hydrocephaly (big heads) not identifiable by external examination who will be more safely born by caesarean (286). With fetal monitoring (which does not have to be continuous) and a good understanding of what the variations in a baby's heart rate mean we are now able to establish how a baby is coping with labour. We can quickly and easily opt for a caesarean section if this becomes necessary. *We have more information available to us than ever before to make a vaginal breech birth a safe viable option. And yet we are performing more caesareans than ever before.* Over the period of time that these advances have been introduced, our babies have not got any bigger. Indeed they are still not quite the size they were in 1958 (286).

The statement "Caesarean is best for baby" belies one of the true certainties in the entire breech debate: that caesarean is worse for mothers' health. It is far more likely that your recovery time will be slower and you will have more potential for complications with a caesarean than with a vaginal delivery. Caesarean section has a mortality rate four times higher than that of vaginal delivery. Wendy Savage expressed her own dissatisfaction with the notion that women should be given the option of elective caesarean section for breech when the evidence does not support this. She went on to describe a case of a woman who had died as a result of severe infection following an elective caesarean section for breech. She said: "At least you want to be sure that the operation was necessary" (286). Although death following caesarean is now an extremely rare occurrence, it is easy to forget that it is major abdominal surgery with all the resulting risks and complications.

The longstanding habit of using forceps and the lithotomy position (on your back with your feet in stirrups), often with an epidural in place, as being the only safe way to conduct a vaginal delivery of a breech baby is similarly non-evidence based. To many of those of us uninitiated in the whys and wherefores of obstetric practice, the lithotomy position and forceps have a bizarre, almost mediaeval, instrument-of-torture-like quality (they don't really do that do they?). It is often the only vaginal breech birth scenario presented leaving many women feeling that an elective caesarean section is infinitely preferable. Although many doctors would tell you that this practice is supported by research, a careful examination of the history of the use of forceps for breech (provided in Chapter 9) suggests that this is not so. The use of forceps for breech is hotly contested in some circles and it could be suggested that an overdependence on forceps and epidurals is precisely the reason some doctors experience vaginal birth as hazardous.

Indeed there are those who argue that the medicalisation of vaginal breech birth is inherently dangerous. Michel Odent has argued that much of the theory he pioneered for active birth (promoting the woman's feelings of safety and privacy, giving birth in a warm, dimly lit comfortable room in an upright position) is even more critical to the success of a vaginal breech birth than a head down one. He argues that he would not "risk" delivering a breech baby in the lithotomy position (see Chapter 9): "It's as if with a breech you are expecting something a little more difficult than the average, so you make it still more difficult artificially – it should be the opposite" (288). Odent even speculates that if it is not possible to find the right conditions, a caesarean may be the best option.[1] The frustrating irony is that in breech birth perhaps more than anywhere else in the world of childbirth, the active birth movement and the obstetric world are pulling in opposite directions. It would seem that good conditions for natural active birth are even more important than with a head down birth, and even more difficult to create. Some women caught in this dilemma opt to have a birth at home but face strong medical censure for so doing. The issue of breech birth at home is discussed in Chapter 11.

Much of the advice given to women carrying breech babies is based on opinion, not evidence. This is not necessarily reason to ignore or dismiss it – opinion is a valid and important part of decision making. However, if you are being advised on the basis of opinion, rather than evidence, you have a right to know. Your own opinion also becomes highly relevant. Indeed, one could argue that the situation is an empowering one – enabling you to team up with your doctor to make a joint decision about what is best for you and your baby.

Sadly, instead of empowerment, there is often an autocratic indifference, or at best a thinly veiled impatience, to any question or opinion you may have. Try to question a caesarean recommending doctor on whether routine elective caesarean for breech is really necessary, or whether routine forceps and epidural are always appropriate in a vaginal breech delivery and you can be left feeling like an irresponsible radical preoccupied with an overvalued idea of vaginal birth, not caring for the safety of her baby and certainly not deserving the privilege of motherhood that awaits you.

For those of you that find yourselves in conflict with your obstetrician about vaginal breech birth, you will not be in terribly radical company. The papers I cite in Chapter 8 supporting vaginal breech birth are generally published in mainstream, establishment, highly respected obstetric and medical journals and written by obstetricians or other doctors. There are eminent obstetricians, some of whom I have interviewed for this book, who believe passionately in the legitimacy of vaginal breech birth as an option for most women carrying breech babies. The problem is, who your doctor is depends largely on where you live – there is a lottery-like quality to the ante-natal care you receive. In the same way as this has been deemed unacceptable in other areas of medicine, I also believe it to be unacceptable in obstetric care. Women should be offered the same opportunities wherever they live and whichever consultant they have.

However, this utopian state of equality of opportunity for all is an ideal and does not help you if you are pregnant and not satisfied with the obstetric care you are getting. The pessimistic reality for some of you is that your options may be limited by your local situation. However, I still feel it is important that you have thought your way through the process and fully understand what is happening to you. This way, even if you have a caesarean that you would have rather not had, you are less likely to spend months and years afterward wondering "What if...?"

---

1. It is important to note that Odent would strongly advocate the use of emergency caesarean (i.e., caesarean after labour has started) as opposed to elective – more on this in Chapter 10.

Information is not always a comfortable possession. One of the things this book does is let you know that certainties about breech birth are much thinner on the ground than many people would have you believe. While this uncertainty may open up new possibilities, it may also leave you feeling anxious and unsure of what to do for the best. One consultant I spoke to gave this as his reason for not sharing the decision making process about a breech birth with a woman. "It would make them terribly anxious," ran his argument, "and women don't want that at the end of their pregnancies." This well intentioned but paternalistic protectiveness is concisely addressed by the late Peter Huntingford.

As a doctor I am well aware that many people would prefer not to take responsibility for medical decisions, but I cannot be certain of this until I have at least offered to share my responsibility with them. (140)

Like him, I believe that you have the right to know what doctors know, and also the limits of their knowledge. You have a right to know where the facts end and opinion begins.

The real concern is that increasingly many junior doctors are emerging from training having little if any experience of vaginal breech birth. The art of vaginal breech birth is dying out. Some would argue the game is already over (287), but others would fiercely maintain that it is a surviving art, albeit a minority one (286). With information about breech birth, women may be more able to seek out second opinions and experienced birth attendants and as they do, send out the message loud and clear to the obstetric and midwifery professions that elective caesarean section as the only option for breech birth is simply not acceptable.

This book is aimed primarily at women carrying breech babies and their partners. However, I also hope the information provided within it will make it important reading for midwives, ante-natal teachers, alternative therapists, and the medical profession.

Wherever and whoever you are, I hope this book is of some value to you. It may or may not make the lead up to your breech birth experience easier, but I hope it enables you to feel as well informed as you possibly can be and equipped to make the difficult decisions that confront you along the way. Above all, I hope it serves to reinforce that this breech baby really is yours and that you have every right to be at the helm, steering your way through the decisions of these last difficult weeks, before you finally meet him or her.

Part One

The What, Why and How Does it Feel?
of Breech

1
What is a Breech Baby?

INTRODUCTION

"Breech" refers purely and simply to the position your baby takes up in the womb. Most babies are vertex, also termed cephalic – they have their heads down ready to engage in your pelvis and pass through the cervix at birth. Breech babies are the opposite – their heads are up and their bottoms are down. Breech literally means "buttocks" and breech is often described as "bottom first". Although many breech babies do have their bottoms as the "presenting part" (i.e., the body part first passing through the cervix in labour), some are feet or foot first, and in rare cases some may be knee or knees first. Different types of breech presentation are described in this chapter.

Breech presentation is not the same as transverse lie, in which the baby is also not head down but is lying across the womb. This book is not directed towards women with transverse babies although part two on turning is relevant to both transverse and breech.

This chapter also covers methods of diagnosing breech babies and the rates of undiagnosed breech births (or those babies not diagnosed as breech until after labour has started).

HOW MANY BABIES ARE BREECH?

Although around a quarter of all babies are breech before 30 weeks of pregnancy, this figure reduces to around 3–4% presenting as breech at term. Chapter 4 gives more detailed information about when most of this turning takes place.

TYPES OF BREECH PRESENTATION

There are various ways of categorising the different types of breech lie and I will try to cover all of them so that you are able to interpret the terms that your medical team is using. If you remain confused by the labels being used ask someone to draw you a diagram of the position your baby is in. The type of breech lie may have implications for your decision about the way you want to give birth so it is important that you know. However, midwife Jane Evans suggests that breech babies may move their legs and change position so do not assume your baby's present position is final (94). The diagnosis of a footling breech in particular is really only one which is appropriate after labour has started as beforehand it is difficult to tell whether a foot or a bottom will present at the cervix.

In an extended or frank breech the baby has its legs extended with its feet up by its ears, almost splinting the body (Figure 1.1). This type of breech is particularly common in first time mothers and is seen as being particularly well suited to vaginal delivery (see Chapter 8 on selection criteria).

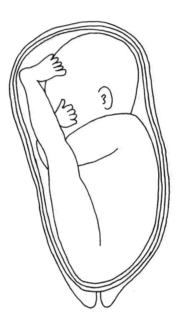

1.1   Extended or frank breech

An extended breech is sometimes also described as an incomplete breech (although the fact that there are various types of incomplete breech make this a somewhat confusing label). In the largest and most recent study of outcomes in breech babies 66.5% of women had extended breeches (127).

In the complete breech (Figure 1.2), the legs are flexed much as they are in a head down/vertex baby. During labour the bottom enters the birth canal first, closely followed by the legs which remain flexed. This is also seen as being a good presentation for vaginal birth. In the study mentioned above, 32.1% of women had complete breeches.

The footling breech may have one or both legs partially or fully extended stretching down below its body, making the presenting part a foot or feet (Figure 1.3). This type of breech is often subdivided into a single or double footling (the former is shown in Figure 1.3). Only 1.4% of breeches were "footling or uncertain" presentation in the study above (127).

Other rarer presentations not illustrated here include a kneeling breech presentation, where one or both knees present to the cervix, or some combination of the above (such as one knee and one foot presenting, or one leg extended up by the ear and the other flexed).

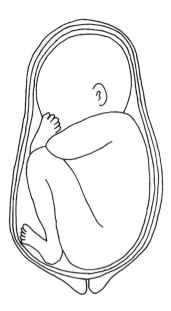

1.2　Complete, full or flexed breech

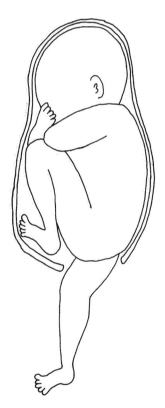

1.3　Footling or incomplete breech

HOW CAN YOU TELL IF A BABY IS BREECH?

The woman's own sensations

A comment that "something is very hard under my ribs" is apparently common, as is the complaint that the area just under the ribs feels bruised after 30 weeks of pregnancy (16). Indigestion may be more common in women carrying breech babies later on in pregnancy because of the greater pressure exerted by the head on the stomach. If your baby gets hiccups, you may notice that you feel the movements near your ribs rather than lower down (16). The location of kicking is a less reliable indicator as, depending on the type of breech you have, the feet may be kicking in the upper or lower part of your womb.

Palpation

Most breech babies are diagnosed by palpation – the process of exploring the baby's position by touch. According to Maggie Banks, a midwife experienced in looking after women with breech babies in New Zealand and author of a book on the subject, there are various signs to look for when palpating a baby that could be breech (16). The key is determining whether the smooth curved shape at the top of the womb can be moved independently of the body. When "ballotted" – gently bounced back and forth between the hands – a head will move independently whereas a bottom will not. If the baby is head down, cupping the baby's bottom in one hand and using gentle forward pressure on the bottom will stimulate the baby to stretch a leg out, which can be felt on the other side of the abdomen.

It is notoriously difficult to distinguish a bottom from a head. One study on the role of palpation stated:

Abdominal palpation for malpresentation [a term which includes breech among other abnormal presentations] has always been an important part of antenatal care. Unfortunately it is a most inexact procedure. Many babies suspected of presenting by the breech, are found to be cephalic when examined by ultrasound and more importantly, palpation sometimes fails to detect the real breech baby. (304)

A midwife mentioned to me the ease with which an occipito-posterior baby (a baby lying with its back to your back) can be easy to confuse with a breech as it is harder to locate the head and buttocks as the limbs present to the front of the uterus where palpation is occurring (69). The heartbeat also comes from a similar place in the two presentations.

In a brief article entitled "Deeply engaged head: is it a breech presentation?" the authors found that over half the women whose breech presentations were not diagnosed until they were in labour had been told their baby's head was deeply engaged in the pelvis at their last examination (191). This study provides a useful caution to any professional diagnosing a deeply engaged head by palpation and also concludes that ultrasound should be used to confirm a baby's presentation accurately.

Ultrasound

Although the use of ultrasound is questioned in some circles (287, 289), there is little doubt of its value in confirming a breech position. You should certainly never have a caesarean section for breech without having had the baby's position confirmed immediately beforehand by ultrasound.

An editorial in the *British Journal of Midwifery* suggests that the failure to detect a breech until labour has started now has more serious implications than it once did as it denies women the opportunity to access external cephalic version (see Chapter 5) late on in their pregnancy if they want to (304). They conclude that ultrasound should be used routinely in late pregnancy to confirm the baby's position.

UNDIAGNOSED BREECH

Rates for undiagnosed breeches vary from as little as 1 in 10 to one third of all breech babies (287). In one study rates of undiagnosed breech were as high as two thirds, though this included a high number of unbooked mothers (those who had not received obstetric care prior to labour starting) (217). Rates also tend to be higher where premature births are included.

Interestingly, studies comparing outcomes of undiagnosed breeches with those diagnosed before labour starts have failed to show any benefit (for mother or baby) for those having the supposed advantage of diagnosis in pregnancy. Indeed one study shows a dramatically higher rate of successful vaginal delivery in the undiagnosed group (42% as opposed to only 11% of diagnosed mothers) (171). This could be for various reasons including the possibility that undiagnosed breeches are likely to be well engaged and therefore well suited to labour, the possibility that the selection criteria applied when a breech is diagnosed unneces- sarily exclude women from a trial of labour (see Chapter 9), the possibility that the woman will not have received the dubious benefit of an interventionist management of her labour (see Chapter 10) and the possibility of a "nocebo effect" (see Chapter 3) – a term coined by Michel Odent referring to the potentially damaging psychological effect of a breech diagnosis on women and profession- als (212).

However, as mentioned above, the key practical advantage to earlier diagnosis is the opportunity to access ECV (external cephalic version – described in Chapter 5). Emotionally too, although the diagnosis of breech in pregnancy can be anxiety inducing and some have argued that the mother is almost better off not knowing (212), there may well be advantages to having time to prepare and adjust to a diagnosis of breech. Meniru and Reginald comment: "the degree of psychologi- cal stress to the mother on the sudden reversal of earlier pronouncements on fetal presentation and delivery plans should not be underestimated" (191).

SUMMARY

Babies are described as lying in the breech position when they have their bottoms and/or feet down towards the mother's cervix and pelvis and their heads up towards the mother's chest and ribs. Although around 25% of babies lie in the breech position at 30 weeks, the vast majority of babies turn, leaving only 3–4% born as breech at term. The three main types of breech presentation are illustrated (extended/frank, flexed/full/complete, footling/incomplete) and other rarer forms of breech presentation described. There are various ways of diagnosing a breech baby including internal cues reported by the mother (such as feeling something hard under the ribs), palpation (external examination by touch) and ultrasound. Ultrasound is by far the most reliable and accurate of these and should always be undertaken if confirmation of the diagnosis is required. It should always be used immediately prior to caesarean section for breech.

Somewhere between 1 in 10 and 1 in 3 breech babies are not diagnosed until after labour has started – and are termed "undiagnosed breeches". Although studies suggest that outcomes are no different for diagnosed and undiagnosed breeches (and that the latter may have higher rates of successful vaginal delivery), the emotional turmoil diagnosis in labour can cause and the inability to access ECV (external cephalic version – see Chapter 5) in late pregnancy need to be taken into consideration.

2
Why are Babies Breech?

INTRODUCTION

The simple answer to "Why is my baby breech?" is "We probably don't know." It is common for people to give you the impression that your baby may be breech because there is something wrong with it. While there may be a problem in a small minority of cases, the vast majority (over 93%) of breech babies are born normal with no congenital abnormality of any kind (93). What follows is a review of the various reasons people have suggested for babies assuming a breech position. However, be warned: you may finish this chapter without an answer to the question of why your baby is breech.

There is no single reason for babies being breech. The underlying causes for breech have exercised minds for many years, with few clear conclusions. The most recent study on the causes of a breech presentation, conducted in 1996, concluded: "Several different maternal and infant characteristics appear to increase risk of breech birth, suggesting that there may be several different biological mechanisms leading to breech birth" (235). One report of an inconclusive study looking at causes for breech commented: "the instances in which a rational explanation for the breech presentation could be found were comparatively few. In the majority of cases, no single cause could be identified."

The uncertainty surrounding the subject helps to explain this rather exasperated conclusion in the *Lancet* in 1940:

> What struck me and still impresses me concerning the etiology [i.e., cause] of breech presentation is that most of these factors which are reputed to be causes, seldom occur. I concluded therefore that either the "cause" is so rare as to be almost a chance coincidence, or that the cause in almost every case is unknown. (303)

Much more recently, reviewers of evidence on the causes of breech birth commented: "Breech presentation has been largely attributed to random occurrence" (19).

Part of understanding why babies are breech involves understanding why most babies lie with their heads down and it is to this that we shall turn first. For many centuries it was believed that all babies sat in the breech position during pregnancy, and then tumbled into a head down position at the end of pregnancy because the head had become "top heavy" and was pulled down by gravity (85). This gravitation theory remained popular until the mid nineteenth century when various sources

15

of evidence refuted it. This included observations that head first birth was normal for most of the animal kingdom, despite the fact that their four legged stance would prevent gravity causing this, and also evidence showing that infants with unusually large heads (hydrocephalic) had a greater tendency to be born breech than infants with unusually small heads (anencephalic) – the opposite to what gravitation theory would predict (85). Further theorising led to the development of the "accommodation theory", which stated that infants moved into the head down position later in pregnancy because it represented the best fit between the baby's body and the mother's uterus (19). Caseaux and Tarnier wrote in 1885 that "the folded condition of the lower limbs is much more voluminous than the head, [and] must naturally lie in the largest cavity, that is towards the fundus [the top of the uterus]" (44). By 1931 Taussig suggested that the process was a combination of maternal and fetal factors: the presence of a normal maternal pelvis and uterus, and a single term fetus with adequate kicking movements resulting in a head down presentation by the end of pregnancy (283). This view (with the exception of a role for the mother's pelvis which is no longer thought to be relevant) is now widely accepted.

For clarity, the factors in the mother and the baby which may lead to breech presentation will be examined separately.

FACTORS IN THE MOTHER INCREASING
THE RISK OF BREECH PRESENTATION

Features of the mother's body

The pelvis

Taussig's suggestion that the maternal pelvis may play a role in causing babies to turn head down is dismissed by Bartlett and Okun as a reason for breech (19). The way the baby presents, they suggest, is settled long before it enters the pelvis, so this is unlikely to have any influence on presentation. To confirm this, two studies in the 1940s reported that women with breech babies had no higher levels of very small pelvises than women with head down babies (297, 316).

However, Maggie Banks suggests that a misshapen pelvis can be a cause for a breech presentation (16). She suggests that previous injury to the pelvis, childhood malnutrition, or use of the oral contraceptive pill during adolescence (before the pelvic cavity has matured fully) can cause a pelvic shape which favours breech, though she does not cite any evidence in support of this. Donald Gibb has also suggested that a small pelvis may prevent a baby's head from settling into a head down position (115).

The uterus

If the baby's position is determined in part by the shape of the uterus, then variations in uterine shape may contribute to breech presentation. However, if the breech presentation were caused only by the shape of the mother's uterus, we might expect to see breech birth in every subsequent pregnancy of a woman who has had one breech baby. In fact, Tompkins (297) found that only 9.4% of women who had their first baby in the breech position went on to have a second breech baby. His review of the literature showed a range of 3.7–10.9% from other studies. More recently, Luterkort et al. reported a higher level of 21% (178). These figures suggest that the chance of having a second breech baby after having had one already lie somewhere between approximately 1 in 20 and 1 in 5. In many cases, though not necessarily all, a uterine shape which favours breech presentation may be due to inherited factors. Cartledge and Hancock presented a fascinating breech family tree in 1942 (see Figure 2.1) (43).

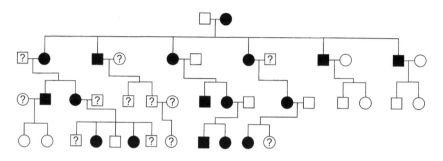

Key
circle = woman
square = man
black   = born breech
white   = born head down
query   = birth position unknown

2.1   A family tree showing inheritance of the tendency to be born breech in one family

Source: Cartledge, L.J. and Hancock, F.Y. Inherited breech presentation. *Journal of Heredity* 33 (1942): 409–10. Reproduced with permission from Oxford University Press.

The tree starts with one breech born woman, whose six children were all born as breech. Of these children, the three daughters went on to have all breech babies. The three sons all married women who had not been born breech and all had head down babies (though the data is not complete for the son's spouses and children). In the next generation, over half of the daughters' children were breech. Unfortunately there was no data on any children the daughters of the sons may have had, preventing us from establishing whether the tendency to have breech babies can be passed down by men to their daughters. Of the total of 29 descendants from this one woman, 16 were born breech, 7 were head down and 6 were unknown. If one examines the female line only, 13 of the 17 children born to women in the family were breech, 1 was head down and 3 were unknown. The authors conclude that the presentation of infants by the breech when it runs in families seems to be due to the presence of a single dominant gene. This means that there is a 75% chance of it being inherited. This gene is likely to determine the shape of your uterus in such a way that it makes it more likely for your baby to decide that a breech position is a better fit than a head down position.

There are features about inherited breeches which differentiate them from other breech babies. Unsurprisingly they are less likely to be successfully turned with external cephalic version (see Chapter 4) (80). They also have better outcomes (i.e. are less likely to have congenital abnormalities) which makes sense given that the cause of the breech position is likely to be related to the shape of the mother's uterus rather than factors in the baby (7).

You should be careful not to leap to conclusions about inheritance however. If your mother or father was breech born, and you were too, this is not sufficient indication to suggest that your baby (and subsequent babies) will be. As we have already seen, most occurrences of breech birth will be due to factors other than inherited ones. Just by chance there will be times when children of breech babies have their own breech babies for unrelated reasons. However, if you have a grandparent who was also breech, and if any of your aunts and uncles were, this increases the likelihood of your baby lying in the breech position due to an inherited tendency.

The uterus shape most often associated with a breech presentation is a bicornuate uterus (see Figure 2.2). "Bicornuate" means literally "having two horns". The head occupies one horn, the legs and feet the other (111).

A similar effect is derived from "uterine septum", a full or partial vertical division of the uterus (see Figure 2.3). In extreme cases there can be a complete vertical division of the uterus. More often it manifests as a heart shaped uterus. The baby will either assume an extended breech position using both sides of the uterus, or if the septum is not too long, the larger space becomes the lower part of the uterus

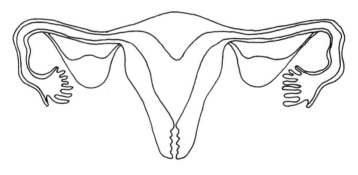

2.2   Bicornuate uterus

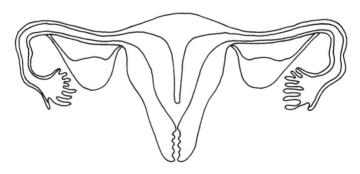

2.3   Uterine septum: a partial division of the uterus

above the pelvis and your baby may find it more comfortable to put its bottom and folded legs here. Two sources I have come across believe the role of uterine septum may be responsible for more breeches, especially non-turnable extended breeches, than generally thought (16, 276). Retained placenta is more common in both of these groups. Both conditions are difficult to spot and may remain undiagnosed throughout your pregnancy.

Banks also points out the role of fibroids growing low in the uterus which can alter the uterine shape and favour a breech presentation (16). These would normally be picked up on an ultrasound scan.

Studies looking at uterine "anomalies" (including unusually shaped uteri and the presence of tumours or fibroids) found that between 28% and 47% of women with uterine anomalies had breech presentations (3, 24, 192). An unusually shaped uterus therefore increases the risk of breech presentation.

Placental location

Placental location was thought to be a cause of breech birth, and was the subject of a paper by Stevenson in 1950 confidently entitled "The principal cause of breech presentation in single term pregnancies" (274). He found a majority of women with breech presentations to have a cornual-fundal placental implantation (in the upper part of the uterus), and this finding was confirmed in a couple of later studies (100, 154), one of which found 72.6% of women with breech presentations to have cornual-fundal implantations, compared to 4.8% of women with head down babies (154). The hypothesis was that the location of the placenta in the upper area of the uterus changed its shape to favour a breech lie. However, Bartlett and Okun (19) have criticised these findings from a pre-ultrasound era and cite a study which used ultrasound to identify placental location in breech babies at 32–33 weeks of pregnancy. No difference was found between babies who later turned to being head down and those who stayed breech.

It has also been suggested that placenta praevia (a placenta implanted in the lower part of the uterus which may be fully or partially covering the cervix) may be causally linked to breech (see Figure 2.4). Placenta praevia may displace the

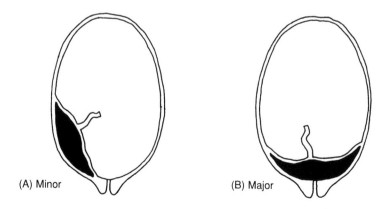

(A) Minor   (B) Major

2.4 Different types of placenta praevia

presenting part from the pelvis and prevent engagement, therefore making the baby's position unstable for longer. Maggie Banks also suggests that placenta praevia changes the shape of the uterine cavity so as to favour a breech presentation (16). However, Rayl et al. found no support for an association between breech and placenta praevia in their large scale study (235) (though this may have been because the number of women with placenta praevia is small).

Amniotic fluid volume
The amount of amniotic fluid, both too little and too much, has been thought to increase the chances of breech birth. Bartlett suggests that too little fluid reduces the baby's ability to move freely enough to turn because the space is more restricted. In contrast, too much fluid means that the baby is not forced to find a stable lie and can move freely right up to the time of birth (19). However, Rayl et al.'s findings suggest that fluid abnormalities may be associated with breech through other factors, rather than directly causally linked, in the case of too much fluid at least (235) (see below).

Bartlett estimates that "mechanical maternal factors" such as those discussed above account for less than 15% of breech births (19).

The impact of previous pregnancies
The higher incidence of breech birth in first pregnancies was first noted by Tompkins (297) in 1946 and is now well recognised (85). This is generally thought to be because in a first pregnancy the baby has less available space to move around because of the uterine and abdominal walls being less stretchy. It is often suggested that the baby simply gets caught in a breech position and finds itself unable to move as the pregnancy goes on. Another possibility emerging in one study was that findings of an association between breech and first pregnancies may be mediated by lower birthweights (see below) (239).

The most recent and large scale study on the causes of breech, conducted by Rayl et al. in 1996 of 3588 breech births in Washington State, also showed that a first pregnancy increases the likelihood of a breech birth (235). They calculated from their data that in comparison with a woman having her first baby, women with one previous birth have a reduction in risk of breech birth of approximately 40% and women with more than one previous birth would have an approximate 64% reduction in risk. They also found that there was a slight elevation of risk in breech birth in women with more than three previous births, which confirms an earlier finding that women with more than five previous full term births have a higher rate of breech presentation (25). This is presumably because the baby remains able to move more freely in its well stretched uterine cavity up to the end of the pregnancy and is not encouraged by the normal constraints of space to find a good fit. However, the increased risk of several previous pregnancies is much less than that caused by a first pregnancy (235).

It has also been observed that mortality in breech babies is lower in first born breech babies than in breech babies born to women who have had previous head down babies. This would suggest that factors in the shape of the womb rather than abnormalities in baby are causing the breech lie (20).

The impact of maternal age

Tompkins also drew attention to the greater tendency of older women in their first pregnancy to have a breech presentation. A recent study found that mothers of breech babies were significantly older than those of head down babies (152). This confirmed Rayl et al.'s findings which showed a smooth, continuous increase in the risk of breech position as the mother's age increased.

Other miscellaneous maternal characteristics

In Rayl et al.'s study black and Filipino women had approximately 60% and 50% decreases in their respective risk of breech birth, compared with white women. This could be related to differences in the shape of the uterus (322), or to differences in characteristics of the babies (see below), or to other causes such as environmental or behavioural factors. They also found a strong association between diabetes (though only diabetes established prior to the pregnancy, not gestational diabetes) and breech birth, with a nearly threefold increase of breech in diabetic women. They link this to decreased fetal movement which has been reported in diabetic pregnancies.

Finally they found that late or no prenatal care was associated with a 30% increase in the risk of breech birth. There may be a range of reasons for this, though it could be linked to losing the opportunity to access attempts at turning the baby using external cephalic version (ECV) (see Chapter 5). Rayl et al. do not mention whether there was an active policy of ECV in the hospitals from which they took their sample.

One study found a significantly higher rate of breech presentation in adult as opposed to teenage pregnancies (8). This could be a combined result of both age and possible lower levels of prenatal care in teenage pregnancies.

Maternal lifestyle factors

Midwife Jean Sutton has written a book called *Understanding and Teaching Optimal Foetal Positioning* and she argues that babies may get into a breech postion early on in pregnancy and, because of our sedentary and inactive lifestyles, find themselves with insufficient space to turn to a head down position later on (279). She views low slung sofas and car seats as particular culprits.

Rayl et al. found maternal smoking during pregnancy to be associated with a 30% increase in risk of breech birth (235). It is likely that smoking operates by reducing the baby's vigour, and therefore its ability to kick itself round (see below, "Factors in the baby").

Psychological factors in the mother

Some people believe that there are emotional reasons for breech presentation. Cheek and Rossi believe that anxious and fearful women have a higher incidence of breech presentation than other women (48). They suggest that the mechanism for this psychological cause of breech is that stress causes tightening of the lower uterine segment which prevents entry and engagement of the baby's head. Tension is the most plausible mediator in any proposed relationship between psychological state and breech presentation.

In discussing this theory, Mehl (190) points to evidence showing that when pregnant mothers are stressed, their babies move around more. He suggests that this could also cause a breech presentation by "preventing the natural setting of the baby's heaviest part usually driven by gravity". However, this line of theorising is based on a misconception of the process by which babies assume a head down position (see the challenge to the gravitation theory at the beginning of this chapter), and as explained later in this chapter, greater movement in the baby should lead to it being less, not more likely to present as breech.

Maggie Banks, a midwife from New Zealand with wide experience of breech birth, comments: "In my own practice I have repeatedly seen the impact of emotional factors on the baby's presentation" (16). She gives two examples, one of which suggests that the breech presentation was caused by the woman's anxiety and tension about a breech birth, and another in which it is suggested that the baby assumed a breech birth in order to be noticed by a busy and preoccupied mother. In both cases the babies turned to being head down when the mothers addressed the apparent psychological cause; accepting the possibility of a breech birth in the former case, and paying the baby attention in the latter. Clearly the difficulty with interpreting such case examples is the very real possibility that these babies may have turned anyway, regardless of their mothers' psychological state.

Lynn Baptisti Richards in her book *The Vaginal Birth After Caesarean Experience* takes the following approach to women carrying breech babies:

> Whenever a woman has a breech baby we can approach this situation with two different attitudes. We can believe that the breech is a signal that something is wrong that needs to be righted, or that everything is just fine and just the way the baby needs to be. I usually try to present both points of view. I ask her what in her life feels upside down, and also ask her to spend some time with her baby finding out what it is that her baby needs from her. Why is it that her baby needs to feel so close to her heart? Why is it that this baby might want to be born sitting down or with his feet on the ground? I find that trying to force the baby to turn around is not usually as effective as helping the woman to direct her energy toward an inwardly safe resolution. Often, once the woman feels safe the baby settles into a safe position – whether that position be vertex or breech. (238)

Gina Lowden develops this idea and explores the concept of a "birth energy" influencing the baby's position:

> Although many care providers would poo-poo the idea of the existence of a "birth energy", the concept may be especially relevant where breech babies are concerned. As birth draws near, a woman's energy generally becomes more focussed "below the waist". For all we know, babies may literally follow their mother's lead – heading to where the "energy" is. A mother who chooses or is forced to stay in her head (for instance one who is working up to the last minute, who is in conflict in her other relationships, or who is unable to turn off the mental gymnastics such as irrational, fearful "what ifs" about the birth) is focussing her energy "above the waist"....If a mother is able to acknowledge

and perhaps dispel her fears, or overcome the difficulties that are causing her world to feel upside down, and "let herself go" into the reality of impending birth and motherhood, then the baby may turn. (176)

Whether or not these ideas make sense to you about your own situation will depend on your attitudes to this kind of theorising. I would sound a word of caution before drawing any conclusions. There are likely to be many women who are busy, preoccupied, stressed and anxious whose babies do not end up in a breech position. The idea of breech birth is highly likely to generate anxiety and tension without this necessarily causing or contributing to breech presentation. Many women become anxious about birth for a wide range of reasons, and this does not cause their babies to be breech. In order to establish whether there is any link between breech presentation and emotional state, research would need to be conducted on a large sample of pregnant women with breech babies to see whether there were any psychological differences between those whose babies turned head down and those whose babies stayed breech. Alternatively one could assess a sample of women, early in pregnancy, prior to breech being diagnosed and see if there were any psychological differences between those who ultimately had breech babies and those who did not. However, such research has not been done, and is probably unlikely to be done.

Evidence that could be used to support the role of psychological factors in causing breech birth comes from the well designed hypnotherapy study described in Chapter 7. More women undergoing hypnosis had babies who turned to head down than women who did not. What is not clear from the study is the degree to which the success was due to the muscular relaxation induced by a hypnotic state which may have acted physically by creating a little more space for the baby to move, or due to the hypnotic suggestions aimed at improving acceptance and psychological well-being about the birth. Either way, success at turning a breech baby does not necessarily mean that the cause has been identified. Releasing muscular tension may encourage a baby to turn but does not mean that the baby was breech in the first place because of tension.

What concerns me about psychological explanations is that they may not always be helpful for the woman. In both of Maggie Banks' cases cited above, addressing the difficulties the women were having was undoubtedly beneficial for them, regardless of whether it was responsible for their baby's turning or not. Equally, seeking a resolution of stresses and anxiety as suggested by Lynn Baptisti Richards and Gina Lowden is likely to improve emotional well-being and preparedness for the birth immeasurably. However, the danger is that suggesting that the baby's position is somehow the mother's fault could serve to increase her anxiety and sense of self-blame unnecessarily especially where the breech lie persists. The causes of breech ultimately remain shrouded in a fair degree of mystery, and if you find the idea that your baby's position is related to your psychological state a persecutory one then you would do better to ignore it. There is little evidence to support it.

FACTORS IN THE BABY INCREASING THE RISK
OF BREECH PRESENTATION

Extended legs

Stabler (272) proposed in 1947 that fetal kicking was key to most babies ending up head down. When the baby's feet are in the lower part of the uterus, even the smallest of kicks will encounter the bony pelvis, a solid surface which enables a kick that is more likely to lead to effective rotation. Once the baby is in the head down position its feet kick ineffectually against the soft uterine and abdominal walls at the top of the uterus, producing little significant movement. Stabler went on to suggest that extended legs were therefore likely to be one clear cause of breech birth. The baby with extended legs kicks in the same part of the uterus as where its head is. It is therefore more likely for its head to get stuck in the upper part of the uterus. In contrast the baby with flexed legs kicks on the opposite side of the uterus to where its head is, making it more likely that its head will end up in the lower part of the uterus. This paper developed the link between extended legs and breech already suggested by Vartan (303) and Tompkins (297). They suggested two other ways in which extended legs and breech might be causally related. The first was that the shape of a baby with extended legs is different to the baby with flexed legs (see Figure 2.5). The baby's bottom is narrower than its head end when the baby's legs are extended, whereas when they are flexed the diameter of the head is smaller.

This makes it a better fit for the baby with extended legs to sit with its head and feet in the roomier, upper part of the uterus. The second reason they advanced for extended legs leading to breech was that the legs splinted the body, making kicking

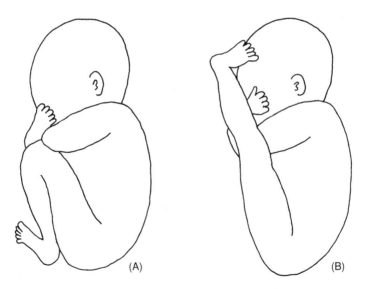

(A)   (B)

2.5   Side view of a baby (A) with legs flexed (the position of most head down babies) and (B) with legs extended (the position of many breech babies)

difficult. More recently, Dunn commented on "the helpless condition of the fetus presenting by the breech with extended legs. The uterus has him in what wrestlers call 'the folding body press'" (85).

If extended legs were a cause of breech presentation, we would expect to see far fewer cases of extended legs in head down pregnancies. Dunn presented precisely this finding in 1976 (85). At 34 weeks, 10% of the head down babies he X-rayed compared to 70% of the breech babies had extended legs. Others have reported 60% of breech babies being born with extended legs, a far higher rate than for head down babies (297, 303).

Of all the causes of breech, it would seem that extended legs accounts for the most cases. However, on the question of what causes extended legs, the literature is disappointingly silent. One study showed that the baby's legs were extended in 74% of first breech pregnancies as opposed to only 55% of second and subsequent breech pregnancies (168), suggesting that a first pregnancy may increase the risk of extended legs. This confirmed previous observations by Tompkins and Stabler, though I have found no-one who has suggested a mechanism for this link. Perhaps the baby with extended legs is making a more efficient use of space by stretching its legs, favoured by the less roomy conditions of a first pregnancy. Further theorising on this is awaited with interest.

It is worth being aware that breech babies who have spent most of their time in the womb with their feet by their ears take a little time to adjust to the roomy conditions of the world after birth. It is quite normal for their legs to continue to move up to their ears, particularly when their clothing and nappy are removed, for several days afterwards.

Congenital abnormalities

The vast majority of serious congenital abnormalities are picked up at 20 week scans (115), so if you had a scan then and all was well, it is unlikely that a congenital abnormality is causing your baby's breech lie. Congenital abnormalities can be defined as malformations or other problems present at birth (but not caused by the birth). They occur three times more often in breech babies as in head down babies. The overall level for breech is 6.3% as opposed to 2.4% for head down babies which includes the full range of mild to severe abnormalities (65). The main way in which congenital abnormalities appear to cause breech presentation is by reducing the baby's ability to kick. The more severely the muscle tone is affected, and the more the abnormality affects the lower limbs, rather than the upper limbs, the more likely the baby is to be breech (19). One example of this emerges from a survey of babies with spina bifida (85). Overall, 38% of babies with spina bifida were born as breech. However, 93% of the subset of spina bifida babies with paralysed legs were born as breech.

Degree of "vigour"

The baby's "vigour", or how much it moves around, even when affected by factors less severe than congenital abnormality, also seems to play a role in causing breech presentation. Babies affected by a whole range of maternal characteristics or behaviour are more likely to present by the breech probably because these factors cause them to kick less. These factors include established maternal diabetes (not gestational) (235), maternal smoking (235), excessive maternal caffeine intake (19), maternal alcoholism and maternal psychotropic drug abuse (19).

A recent study found differences in the motor function of 90 normal breech babies at birth and six weeks compared to head down babies of the same gender and mode of delivery (20). These differences were unrelated to the mode of delivery. At 18 months three of the breech babies were diagnosed with neurological abnormalities, all of whom were born in the caesarean group. Another similar study on reflexes found differences between breech and head down babies' movements at birth, 6 weeks, 3 and 5 months (21). This lends further credence to the idea that breech babies may be lying in the breech position because of differences in their motor ability.

Bartlett also reports evidence from studies of babies with "increased motor competencies". Babies of black African descent are known for this increased vigour. They tend to move around more and do not settle in a stable position until later in pregnancy than caucasian babies. They are at least half as likely to be born breech as caucasian babies (19, 235). This suggests that the baby's ability to kick itself round is of considerable importance and in the case of black African babies has a strongly protective effect against breech birth.

Prematurity

Dunn reported that 25% of the premature babies in his study were born breech (as opposed to 7% of the full term babies), nearly a fourfold increase (85). The most common explanation for this is that premature babies have had more space to move around in and have therefore had no need to assume a stable position. Rayl et al. found that up to 37 weeks, there was a 9% reduction in the chances of having a breech baby as every week of pregnancy went by (235). From 40 weeks, for those babies not yet born, there was little change, suggesting that if the baby is going to turn, it will have done so by this point.

Birthweight

Although birthweight is linked to gestational age, Rayl et al. found there to be a direct link between reduced birthweight and increased risk of breech (235). They comment: "Larger fetuses may be more likely to be forced into the vertex [head down] position in the uterus, whereas smaller fetuses may be less constrained to a specific position." A larger baby may be forced to find the best fit available. One older study has reported high birthweight to be "an accepted cause of breech presentation" (154). However, Rayl et al. found high birthweight to have a protective effect (235).

Another study found small size for gestational age to be associated with breech presentation (239). The authors suggest that the association they also found between breech and female sex can also be explained by the lower birthweight of girls.

Bartlett reports that reduced growth predates breech presentation, suggesting that there is nothing about breech presentation per se which inhibits growth (19). She goes on to suggest that reduced growth may be caused by problems in the baby's or the placenta's circulatory system which could also lead to the baby being less able to kick itself round to a head down position. Luterkort et al. (178) reported that the breech babies in their sample were small for their age and suggest that "a moderate intrauterine growth retardation" may be involved in causing some cases of breech.

Other abnormalities

Various studies suggest that some breech babies may be in some way different to cephalic babies. Although these differences would not be classed as abnormalites as such, they may give clues as to the reasons for breech presentation. One study found that breech babies exhibited more "behavioural state transitions" (152). These transitions appear to have been between low and high heart rate patterns, though how this relates to breech presentation is not altogether clear.

Michel Odent suggests that an immature vestibular system may be responsible for some cases of breech, by affecting a baby's sense of balance and orientation (212).

Twins and multiple births

Breech birth of at least one child is significantly higher in a multiple pregnancy, although figures are only available for twins. Estimates of 34% (85) to 40% (16) of at least one twin being breech have been reported. This tenfold increase over singleton pregnancies is likely to be accounted for mainly by:

1. the different shape of uterine cavity within which each twin has to accommodate itself
2. the increased rate of pre-term delivery in twins
3. less space meaning that the baby may get stuck in a breech position early on and be less able to turn to head down.

SUMMARY

Babies assume a head down position through a combination of their kicking and their overall shape fitting best in this position. There are likely to be many different reasons for breech birth rather than a single cause. Some of these reasons are related to the mother and some to the baby. Approximately 1 in 10 women go on to have a second baby in the breech position after having a first breech baby, suggesting that most of the causes are related to a specific pregnancy or specific baby. The most likely reasons for at least some breech births are as follows:

1. the shape of the mother's uterus, likely to be due to inherited factors or fibroids within the uterus
2. a first pregnancy (probably because there is less room for the baby to turn to a head down position as the uterine and abdominal walls are less stretchy than in subsequent pregnancies and the baby may get stuck in a breech position)
3. extended legs in the baby (probably because the baby's overall shape is different from that of a baby with flexed legs and its kicking is less effective)
4. congenital abnormalities in the baby (often because the baby is less able to kick itself round)

5. prematurity (probably because the baby has not yet found a stable lie)
6. low birthweight (probably because the baby has more space to move around in and is not forced into a head down position)
7. multiple births (probably because of the increased rate of prematurity, the different shape of the uterine cavity each baby has to accommodate to and the lack of room).

3
The Wrong Way Up?
The Emotional Impact of Breech

INTRODUCTION

The news that your baby is breech and likely to remain that way is often met with alarm. It is also often a situation that feels very isolating – the fact that breech babies make up only 3% of babies born means that you are unlikely to come across another parent of a breech baby during your pregnancy. In this chapter women who have been kind enough to contact me talk about their breech experiences. Everyone's breech experience is unique, but there are also many common themes that emerge. I hope this chapter provides at least some material that you can relate to and reduces somewhat any isolation you may be feeling.

"There is little doubt", my consultant said to me, "that nature did not intend babies to be born this way." So started the persistent message that my baby was the wrong way up. The medical literature reinforces this view with breech commonly being described as an "error of orientation" (92) or a "malpresentation" (304).

For women who have not had previous breech babies and don't come from families where breech birth is common, the shock of the diagnosis is often immense. Some women will have been told their baby is in the breech position from early on. However, there is rarely concern expressed at this early stage because so many breech babies turn as pregnancy progresses. The likelihood of your baby being one of the 3% of babies born as breech seems so minute (these things always happen to other people after all) that there seems little point in planning for a breech birth. Even if you are willing to take the possibility seriously, you will probably be surrounded by people who are reluctant to engage in a discussion of your options (anxiety inducing and uncomfortable as this may prove to be) and prefer to provide reassurance that your baby is bound to turn. In this sense, forewarned is not really forearmed, as women still have to undergo the transition from believing that a normal head down birth is probable once their baby has assumed the right position, to accepting the likelihood of a breech birth.

Often the issue of when to stop trying to turn your baby and start planning for the birth is not an easy one. The process of simultaneously holding in mind two opposing outcomes can be difficult.

I wished that someone would just say to me – "Right, if your baby was going to turn it would have done by now so you can now devote yourself 100% to

29

planning for the birth." It was difficult living with the uncertainty, and sometimes my efforts to help the baby turn just felt so futile.

Anne Catt, who published her story of the birth of her daughter Sadie in the National Childbirth Trust (NCT) journal *New Generation* described this process thus:

We knew that the second baby was in the breech position from early on. At first I remained calm, convinced that the baby would turn and my home birth could be assured. But by 34 weeks I began to have my doubts. Exercises, homeopathy, acupuncture, positive thinking – I tried them all to no avail. At a hospital visit at 37 weeks, I was told that the baby was still breech, too small, and there was not enough fluid. I had to be monitored and scanned....I thought they were going to open me up there and then. What a palaver. I couldn't stop crying. (46)

Others will have the news dropped like a bombshell out of the blue in the last month or so of their pregnancy. Kath found out her baby, Josh, was breech two weeks before he was born:

[The diagnosis] only happened because I had a scan for high blood pressure and the person doing the scan said "It's still breech." I said "What do you mean 'still'?" as I had always been told that it was cephalic and even been told in the last couple of weeks that the head was engaged. I was really shocked at the news and to be honest I wasn't sure what it really meant to me.

Fran found out that her first baby, Rosie, was breech at 38 weeks after a normal pregnancy. "I was immediately re-defined as 'high risk' and given appointments for scans, pelvimetry and to see the consultant. I went home and wept copiously."
    The grief of adjusting to a diagnosis of breech is palpable in many of the accounts I have come across. For so many women, as they start on the uphill struggle of information gathering, opinion seeking and agonising, there is a sense of being robbed of the last final weeks of happy anticipation, relaxation and preparation, and a feeling of any prospect of a normal birth evaporating. Joanne who found out her son, James, was breech at week 37 and was offered an elective caesarean at week 38, described her reaction:

I was upset as all my plans for the birth were turned upside down, I was still at work, and I also felt strongly that I wanted my baby to arrive when he was ready, not when somebody said he should.

Vanessa, whose daughter Poppy was born by caesarean said "I desperately wanted a water birth so I felt disappointed in myself."
    Women often describe feeling very alone during this time. Helen, whose first daughter Caitlin was diagnosed breech at 32 weeks, said: "Going to ante-natal classes at this time seemed to upset me more as all the talk of natural birth seemed

not to be valid for me any more." An experience intended to generate mutual support can feel alienating and ante-natal classes often heighten this by brushing over the topic of breech. "It was only referred to as something you hoped wouldn't happen", one woman told me. The profound sense of difference experienced by couples carrying a breech baby is described by Andrew, whose wife went on to have two breech babies. However, he recalls becoming aware of this issue in an ante-natal class before they knew that their first baby was breech:

I have a vivid memory of being in a large Victorian room at Queen Charlotte's where a doctor was listing various pain relief options, all of which seemed to belong to a previous era as far as we were concerned. She then referred to having a breech baby, and I could have sworn a large spotlight focussed on this quivering couple huddled together at the back. Like a judge she delivered a verdict which condemned these poor parents to a list of procedures and options which made the rest of us grateful that we were normal!
Of course it didn't work out like that.

Michel Odent talks of a diagnosis of breech having a "nocebo effect". He suggests the nocebo effect occurs when "health professionals cause more harm than good by interfering with belief systems, imagination and fantasy life" (212). The diagnosis of breech is often presented with considerable anxiety. "High risk" labelling by professionals can be reinforced by the woman's own feelings of fear generated by a "folk anxiety" about breech (see Introduction). Vanessa's anxiety was worsened by her consultant: "I wanted to know what was wrong with my baby. My consultant scared me on several occasions making me think there could be something wrong with her hips or legs." Beatrice had been initially relaxed when finding out that her daughter, Teri, was breech. "My mother's light hearted descriptions of me bobbing up and down in the womb before a normal delivery helped keep everything in perspective. But if I was unfussed before, the specialist changed all that." Beatrice underwent a painful and unsuccessful ECV attempt and was left feeling "terrified of the horror of just getting it out anyhow, anywhere".

Jenny, whose first baby, Natasha, was breech and who subsequently counselled other women with breech babies through the NCT, said: "In my experience being breech conjures up a frightening scene." This scene is often drawn in detail by the medical profession: the birth must take place in the lithotomy position (on your back with your feet held wide apart in stirrups), using forceps with an episiotomy (a cut to the perineum – the flesh between the vagina and the anus), with an epidural. Or you can have an elective caesarean section. The choice is often offered grudgingly and with a distinct lack of objectivity. Fran describes the conversation she had with her consultant:

I was offered two options by my consultant. My pelvis was deemed "just about okay" and I could, since I seemed to be "that sort of woman" have a go at a vaginal delivery – so long as it was with an epidural and forceps. However, if I was his wife, he would recommend an elective caesarean.

Alternatively you may not be offered a choice at all and simply be booked in for a caesarean section. Wendy Savage described the appalling treatment received by a 19-year-old single parent when she tried to question this approach:

[The policy of elective caesarean section for breech] had been explained to her by the senior registrar and the following week she had asked him whether she could just try labour and see how it went. She described how he turned to her and said scathingly "You can't have listened to a word I said last week"....Nine months later she was still depressed and blaming herself for not having stood up to the arrogant young man who had prevented her from trying to deliver her baby the way she wanted to. (251)

Often the very manner in which the conversation is held is disempowering. Jenny recalls the way in which her options were presented to her:

I was given a pelvic X-ray "to see if there was sufficient space for the baby to be born vaginally". I was then told (lying flat on my back with my dress around my neck) that there was and that I would be given an epidural and episiotomy and that my baby would be delivered by forceps! When I asked what my options were, I was told that the alternative was a caesarean section. Any other course of action would require my signature taking full responsibility for my actions. That made me angry and scared for the well being of my baby.

Chapter 13 addresses the issue of disclaimer signing. You are not, in fact, legally obliged to sign anything in spite of what you may be told.

The feeling of being hemmed in and wanting to retort "neither of the above" to the two options presented is common. Women often report developing frenzied information seeking behaviour. Charlotte whose baby, Ellie, was diagnosed breech at 30 weeks started her research immediately. "My main line of attack was to read everything possible. Every time I went into a bookshop I raided the baby books and looked up 'breech baby'." But these often feel woefully inadequate. Vanessa points out: "There were only tiny little articles in birth books and one leaflet that was useless." Even midwives, who are often perceived to be more supportive than doctors may not help much. Helen said: "the midwives were very good and kind but were not very proactive in directing me to other information sources; they basically took the hospital's line but 'understood' my distress". She continued:

All in all I came out of the experience feeling that I just hadn't been able to get the information I'd needed to make proper informed decisions. I'd felt roller-coastered and bullied, and I felt that if people hadn't bombarded me with scare stories I could have resisted the temptation to be upset long enough to do more thorough research. The scare stories also made me think I had no real time for the research or to do much anyway. I just wished I'd known and read more about the options for breech delivery earlier in my pregnancy.

The burden of making decisions at such a late stage is often overwhelming. There can be few more emotive subjects than the safest way to bring your baby into the world when that baby is growing and moving inside you, and the anxiety and distress this generates permeates the whole decision making process. Opinions and anecdotes creep out of the woodwork and before you know it you may be surrounded by a mass of conflicting stories and advice. It can be particularly hard when people close to you react differently to the situation and can be a real challenge for a relationship where your initial reactions place you in conflict with one another.

Many women come to accept the situation, some with more ease than others. Indeed, for many women this process of acceptance is no major challenge. Paula, who was herself a breech baby, was unsurprised at the news early in her pregnancy that her daughter was breech: "I just casually smiled at my consultant and said 'Yes I know'." Ros managed to maintain a broad perspective on being told her baby was breech: "I felt fine as I was happy that the baby was okay and I didn't feel that breech was that big a problem – there could have been much worse problems."

Clearly one determinant of your reaction is how you feel about caesarean section. Anne was not troubled by the news that her daughter was breech.

I was actually quite relieved that Rebecca was a breech, because I believed that I would have a caesarean section – all my nursing/doctor friends thought I was lucky. Some of my non-medical friends thought that I wasn't going to experience a "real" birth (!) but I didn't really care.

Greta said that initially she "was very happy because I thought that would mean a caesarean section", though she added: " – pain free I thought, naive as I was".

Some of the women who wrote to me reported that the sense of feeling caught between a "rock and a hard place" was liberated by seeking a second opinion. The whole issue of a third option – seeking care that will allow you to have a trial of labour using natural active birth techniques – is addressed in detail in Chapter 12. Some women were lucky enough to find this at their local hospitals and others had to go through the upheaval of transferring their care to a different hospital. Others employed independent midwives.

Anne Catt described her independent midwife, Mary Cronk, well known for her experience with breech births, as "a gale of fresh air" (46). Mary's position on breech is that "Breech is not an abnormal presentation, just unusual." What is powerful about this distinction is that is takes us away from thinking that there is something wrong with our babies and encourages us to simply think of them as lying in a different way.

Indeed the irony is that in any other situation our breech babies would be considered to be the right way up. Few of us would consider spending any length of time upside down, and in my brighter moments I decided that my baby was showing an impressive maturity by preferring to have his head up! Trying to positively construe our baby's presentation may be the first step in preparing for the decisions that lie ahead. In the words of Gina Lowden:

If the baby…remains steadfastly in the breech position, then often the most positive position for the mother to take is that her baby, by whatever unfathomable, primal process, had chosen to be born this way. Having accepted this, the mother is much more free to make decisions about what she feels is the best way for her baby to be born. (176)

Whatever decisions you finally make (or are made for you – breech babies often turn up early, pre-empting any careful planning), it is important to remember that you are not alone. Chapter 12 includes more on peoples' decision making and birth outcomes which may help you to feel less isolated. It is important to seek support where you can. If your local services are not providing it you can contact the Association for Improvements in Maternity Services (AIMS). Many independent midwives are also willing to talk your situation through with you even if you are not planning to engage them as a birth attendant. Both independent midwives and AIMS may be able to put you in touch with other women who have had breech babies. The process of carrying and having a breech baby cannot fail to have an impact upon you emotionally and this can sometimes be profound. A handful of women have described the experience as "life changing". Some have become active birth campaigners or NCT advisers. Another trained to be a midwife as a result of her baby being breech. For those of you who feel that a positive outcome is unlikely beyond giving birth to a healthy baby and that breech is simply a stress to be endured, it is important to keep the longer term view. Although birth regrets can persist long after babies have arrived in the world, it is unlikely that the stress will ever feel as intense as it does in the final weeks of your pregnancy.

SUMMARY

The emotional impact of finding out your baby is breech is an individual experience but common themes emerge in many women's accounts. Shock, grief, and disappointment as hopes for a normal birth seem dashed are common.

Women/couples often feel isolated and different and ante-natal classes can sometimes heighten this feeling of loneliness. Fear, both that there may be something wrong with the baby and of the options for the birth, is also commonly experienced and can be worsened rather than helped by the medical profession's response to breech birth. There is often a feeling that there is not enough time or available information to properly think through the issues involved and make the decisions that are right for you personally. Some women come to accept their situation without too much difficulty and this can be made easier if you have positive feelings about caesarean section. For many women, the whole journey of carrying and giving birth to a breech baby is a major stress which needs to be endured and moved on from as quickly as possible. For others there can be positive and life changing aspects to the experience. Either way the experience is unlikely to leave you unaffected in some way. But do remember – you are not alone!

Part Two
Turning Breech Babies

4
An Introduction to
Turning Breech Babies

INTRODUCTION

This chapter does not demonstrate specific techniques to help your baby to turn. This is covered in detail in Chapters 5 and 7. It aims to raise general issues associated with turning. It covers spontaneous turning – in essence what is likely to happen if your baby is left to its own devices with no effort on your part to turn it. It also discusses some of the general issues of turning such as when to do it, which techniques to choose, how to tell if your baby has turned and why you might or might not want to embark on turning attempts.

SPONTANEOUS TURNING

The vast majority of breech babies turn to the head down position during pregnancy. Approximately 20–30% of babies are in the breech position at 25–26 weeks, 10–15% at 30–32 weeks, while only 3–4% are breech at birth (132, 133, 255).

A significant percentage of the breech babies of pregnant women reading this book will turn before 40 weeks, despite the fact that, having been diagnosed as breech at 36 weeks, many are led to believe that their fate is sealed: "At no point did anyone at the hospital say what my GP did tell me – that there was still plenty of time for the baby to turn by itself" (179). One woman reported the view of her very experienced midwife: "Our own seventy-five year old grand midwife pooh-poohed our consternation. She said that the baby would turn, that sometimes they turn right before the birth, even during labour" (234). However, most of the turning that is going to take place happens before 36 weeks. This is because the baby has less and less room to move around as pregnancy nears its completion.

There are various factors which make a baby more or less likely to turn. Figure 4.1 shows the results of some research monitoring 310 breech babies identified at 32 weeks (314).

The study showed that women who had had at least one baby before, but never had a breech birth, were dramatically more likely to experience spontaneous turning than anyone else. This high rate of turning persisted even at 36–37 weeks when 25% of these babies turned. The group who were least likely to experience spontaneous turning were those who had had at least one previous breech baby. This is probably due to some special characteristic of the mother's uterus or abdominal cavity (see Chapter 2 for causes of breech presentation). Women having their first babies had somewhat higher levels of turning, although this reduced dramatically towards the end of the pregnancy. This is probably due to the particularly

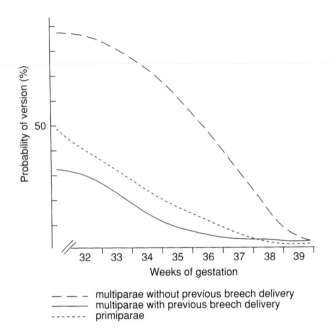

4.1   Likelihood of spontaneous turning during pregnancy in three different groups of mothers

Source: Westgren, M., et al. Spontaneous cephalic version of breech presentation in the last trimester. *British Journal of Obstetrics and Gynaecology* 92 (1985): 19–22. Copyright © 1985. Reprinted with permission from Elsevier Science.

taut muscles of the uterus and abdomen in women having their first babies, creating even less room for manoeuvre as 40 weeks is approached.

The study also showed that babies whose legs were flexed were very significantly more likely to turn around than babies with extended legs (see Table 4.1). The reasons for the lower turning rates of babies with extended legs are discussed in Chapter 2.

Table 4.1   Impact of baby's leg position on turning

Baby's leg position	Persistent breech	Turned spontaneously
Legs flexed at the knees	27 (20%)	92 (52%)
Legs extended	106 (80%)	85 (48%)
Total	133	177

Source: As Figure 4.1. Copyright © 1985. Reprinted with permission from Elsevier Science.

The conclusion seems to be that if you have had children before and none of them were breech born you are less likely to need to plan for a breech birth than other women carrying breech babies. Anyone carrying a breech baby with extended legs is probably more likely to have a breech birth. Anyone who has had one or more breech babies is much more likely to have a breech birth. What this means for your efforts to help the baby to turn, however, is not clear. There is evidence that the same factors that make your baby more likely to turn on its own also facilitate the success of turning attempts such as external cephalic version (ECV) (see Chapter 5). One could equally take the view that if your baby is more likely to turn on its own you may not wish to work so hard at the turning process. As with everything else in this book, it is your decision.

WHICH TURNING TECHNIQUE TO CHOOSE

There are a range of techniques available to help babies turn which are described in Chapters 5 and 6. Some are practised by specialists and others by you. It is important to clarify that attempting to turn your own baby by firmly massaging or pushing it round is not advised and could be dangerous. Techniques which can be safely practised by you tend to involve alternative therapies or exercises.

Some techniques are evaluated rigorously (e.g., ECV), others show promising results in small studies (e.g., acupuncture, positioning, hypnotherapy), and others are based on encouraging anecdotal accounts or techniques that people have argued should work. Some may have possible risks associated with them, while others seem to be free of side effects and may even have other positive spin offs such as increased feelings of relaxation and well-being. While you have a right to access the option of ECV on the NHS, the other techniques should really be employed according to what makes most sense to you, and how much time, energy and, in the case of many of the alternative therapies, money, you wish to devote to trying to turn your baby.

WHEN TO HELP YOUR BABY TO TURN

Currently, it is generally recommended that the time to start encouraging babies to turn in earnest is around 36–37 weeks. There are broadly no inherent problems with trying to turn the baby before this time – it may in fact be easier to turn as the greater space in the womb gives more freedom of movement. However, earlier in pregnancy the baby is both much more likely to turn spontaneously if left to its own devices, and much more likely to turn back to being breech again even if it does turn spontaneously. In the case of ECV there may be risks associated with earlier attempts (see Chapter 6 for a discussion of earlier ECV). It is for this reason that you are unlikely to be offered ECV, certainly on the NHS, before 37 weeks.

If you have the time and inclination, there seems little harm in trying any of the alternative therapies and other techniques mentioned in Chapter 7 earlier than 37 weeks. Acupuncture often starts well before 37 weeks with one study including women at only 28 weeks. Yehudi Gordon, a consultant obstetrician who supports the use of acupuncture in cases of breech, argues for the benefits of having it far earlier than 37 weeks (123). The crawling technique described in Chapter 7 is recommended for all pregnant women to help the baby into a better position for birth, so is probably worth practising as soon as you find out your baby is breech. Midwife Alice Coyle recommends a range of optimal fetal positioning techniques to all the women in her care (including lying on the left side and sitting with the legs apart and leaning forward) from 32 weeks (69).

HOW CAN YOU TELL IF YOUR BABY HAS TURNED?

If you are going to make efforts to turn your baby, you want to make very sure you do not continue once it has turned. Some women report feeling their baby turning clearly as is the case in these two examples: "I felt this turning sensation and when I went for a check up the doctors told me the baby's head was engaged" and "I felt the hardness of the baby's head moving down the wall of my uterus and sure enough, next morning there were tiny kicks in my ribs" (234). The second woman clearly had a flexed breech as when the baby turned she changed from feeling kicks in her pelvis to feeling kicks in her ribs. Women carrying extended breeches are likely to feel kicks around their ribs and upper part of their uterus even when the baby is breech.

Babies may turn at night, perhaps encouraged to do so by your relaxed muscles. Even if you do not feel your baby turn, you may be aware that your body feels different. Maggie Banks says of women carrying breech babies that: "A comment that 'something is very hard under my ribs' is common as is the complaint of a specific area under her ribs feeling bruised when she is more than thirty weeks gestation" (16). She also describes the way that any hiccups in a breech baby may be felt in the upper part of the uterus, under the ribs. Clearly any change in the location of these movements or sensations may be a sign that the baby has turned, even if you haven't felt it do so.

One study on ECV in Africa decided to train women in self-assessment of their baby's position to pick up on babies turning back to breech after successful ECV (270). Women were taught by a health professional to feel their stomachs gently (palpation) and taught the difference between the feel of a head and a bottom. The study was successful and the authors commented "The ability of women to suspect a non-cephalic (i.e., a return to breech) presentation was surprisingly good." Some women who have carried breech babies might be tempted to suggest that the authors' surprise is a little patronising, given that the woman has the benefit of internal bodily cues to assist her diagnosis as well as palpation. The study is nevertheless a good one. Unfortunately this process of involving women in their own care has little precedent in this country's recent obstetric history. However, if you are interested in improving your own ability to identify your baby's position and have a supportive doctor or midwife, you could ask them to show you how. Maggie Banks' book on breech includes a detailed section on palpating a breech baby, intended for midwives, which uses diagrams to help the reader differentiate between a breech and a head down position (16).

Banks warns against doing an internal examination to diagnose a breech in the non-labour situation. In addition to the harm that this could cause, she also points out that with extended breeches, a bottom can feel just as firm as a head, leaving the examiner none the wiser (16). However, Wendy Savage disagrees, arguing that an experienced practitioner can feel a clear difference between a breech and a head down baby (252).

Unfortunately, there are many tales of experienced health professionals getting it wrong, both in the failure to identify a baby in the breech position, and identifying a breech when the baby is in fact cephalic (304). One study observed that the failure to identify a breech often occurs when the position is misdiagnosed as a deeply engaged head. They suggest that careful palpation is undertaken in such circumstances and that access to an ultrasound scanner is of great importance (191). An ultrasound scan is the most reliable way to confirm your breech diagnosis. Indeed, you probably shouldn't be making serious plans for a breech birth until you have had a scan done, ideally at 36–37 weeks (304). If you are planning to have an elective caesarean section, you should always have a scan immediately before it to ensure that the baby is still breech.

POSITIONS TO FACILITATE ENGAGEMENT FOLLOWING TURNING

If you are sure that your baby has turned, you first need to establish that its head down position is a good one for labour, i.e., with the head flexed, and lying well (check this with your midwife). If you are told that this is indeed the case, it is sensible to promote engagement of the head, both to reduce the chances of turning back again and to prepare for the birth. This involves doing the opposite of the positioning methods to encourage turning: you are trying to encourage the head into the pelvis. Regular squatting is probably the most effective. You may want to empty your bladder first to minimise discomfort. You may wish to continue crawling (as recommended earlier to encourage an anterior position) but may want to precede and follow crawling with a few minutes of squatting to make sure that the head is well down. If your baby is not in a good position you may wish to follow the advice given in Jean Sutton's book, *Understanding and Teaching Optimal Foetal Positioning* (279) (details are given in the Further Reading section at the end of this book).

WHY HELP YOUR BABY TO TURN?

Some would say that anything you can do to prevent a breech birth, be it vaginal or caesarean birth is worth trying. One author points out that if turning is successful, it "relieves both mother and obstetrician of the dilemma of choosing between a vaginal or abdominal delivery" (139). If you are planning an elective caesarean for breech, attempting to turn the baby so that you can have a vaginal delivery with a head down baby could save you from the maternal risks associated with caesarean (see Chapter 12). For many the sense that there is something active that can be done helps to keep their spirits buoyant through the last difficult weeks: "It certainly made me feel less anxious and less helpless to have something positive to do" (179).

However, Wendy Savage, a great believer in the safety of vaginal breech birth for most women carrying breech babies, points out: "If you say to a woman 'well I'm going to turn your baby round because it's so much better to have it head first' what does that do to her confidence in having a vaginal breech birth?" (252). One woman approaching the birth of her second breech baby said: "To go into hospital and have ECV would have medicalised the whole thing and brought in the idea that things had gone 'wrong' and needed correcting." Certainly if you have a trial of labour planned with an experienced birth attendant, there are those who would argue that there is no need to try turning the baby.

Some women have a sense of fatalism about their baby being breech which can give rise to a feeling that there is little that can or should be done to change its position. Maggie Banks describes the range of factors which may influence a woman's decision about which techniques, if any, you decide to try:

> Her comfort with the various suggestions will depend on her health, fitness and her spiritual and religious beliefs. Her general feeling about how important, or unimportant, it is to have her baby come head down will also have an impact on her choice as to whether she will try to turn the baby. (16)

Ultimately which turning techniques you use, if any, will depend both on your feelings about your baby being breech and on your views about the turning techniques described in the next two chapters.

SUMMARY

Many breech babies turn spontaneously, leaving only 3–4% of babies still in the breech position at birth. If you have already had one or more baby that was not in the breech position, or if your baby has its legs flexed rather than extended, your baby is more likely to turn to being head down before the birth. It is generally recommended that attempts to turn your baby should start around 37 weeks, but with many of the alternative techniques there is no particular reason to wait if you want to try them earlier than this. You should not attempt to turn the baby yourself by using any force as this can be dangerous. It is worth having the baby's position confirmed, either by an experienced professional, or preferably using ultrasound. If you decide to try to help your baby to turn there are a range of techniques to choose from, described in Chapters 5 and 6. Which technique you choose, if any, is entirely up to you.

5
External Cephalic Version (ECV)

INTRODUCTION

External cephalic version is a technique used by professionals to turn breech babies to a head down position. This chapter tells you what to expect if you undergo ECV, gives a brief historical overview of the technique, discusses reasons why you may not be suitable for ECV (contraindications), looks at the risks and drawbacks of the procedure and the reported success rates. The current status of ECV is discussed, reasons that you may not be offered it given, and some thoughts offered on what to do if you are not offered ECV and you want it.

WHAT IS ECV?

External cephalic version means literally turning (version) the baby to a head down (cephalic) position by means of manual manipulation outside the body (external). It is normally done in hospital, almost always on an out-patient basis, usually by a consultant (though Johanson states that there is no reason why specialised midwives and registrars should not learn to undertake the procedure (145)).

WHAT HAPPENS WHEN YOU HAVE ECV?

The procedure should be explained to you in full, including the rationale, likely success and possible risks of the procedure. Do not assume that this explanation will be given to you automatically – it is not unheard of for a doctor to ask his/her patient to hop up on the examining couch during a routine ante-natal check and forge into ECV without any discussion. Do ask if there is anything that you want to know first. Apart from your basic right to have the procedure explained adequately, the knowledge will help you to feel less anxious and better able to relax (which may contribute towards a successful outcome).

An ultrasound scan is normally carried out beforehand to check the position of the placenta, assess the amniotic fluid volume, confirm the breech position, determine the position of the baby's head, back and limbs, ensure the absence of the cord around the baby's neck, and check for any abnormalities in the baby which would make even a head down vaginal birth complicated. There is little reason for having ECV if you need to have an elective caesarean section for reasons other than breech. A baseline nonstress test should also be done to confirm the baby's well-being using cardiotocography (CTG). This involves monitoring the baby's heart rate for a period of time before the start of ECV.

If your blood group is rhesus-negative, an antibody screen should be carried out prior to and within seven days of your ECV appointment (139). You should be given anti-D immunoglobin (in case of the unlikely occurrence of a bleed of your baby's blood into your blood (which you are unlikely to notice (108) following ECV) (203).

Many doctors, particularly in the UK, carry out ECV in ante-natal clinics, though this should always be in a hospital where there are facilities for offering emergency caesarean section, if necessary. The risk of emergency caesarean section necessitated by fetal distress following ECV is very small at under 1% (145) (2 of 356 version attempts in one study (141)), but some doctors take it sufficiently seriously to perform ECV in the operating theatre and ask their patients to fast beforehand (145, 189).

Some doctors will use a "tocolytic agent" – a medication to relax the uterus, which is injected into your arm before the procedure starts. The drugs most commonly used belong to a group called beta-sympathomimetics and tend to be one of the following: ritodrine, hexoprenaline, terbutaline or salbutomol. If the uterus remains tense after a standard dose, a second dose may be used as long as you experience no significant side effects (203). Possible side effects are described in the next chapter.

You will be asked to lie down and relax as much as you can. Most of the time the procedure will be undertaken with you flat on your back, although suggestions have been made for side lying positions in some cases (134, 203). This is worth considering if you are liable to develop hypotension (low blood pressure which often makes you feel faint or dizzy) when lying on your back or find it uncomfortable and not conducive to relaxation. One report of a case of successful ECV describes lying the woman on an ironing board inclined against a bed, with her head nearest the floor. This tilted the pelvis and the woman lay in this position for 20 minutes beforehand "to allow the baby to float more freely in the womb" (234). Another study reported the use of pillows to tilt the pelvis (139), while another tilted the entire bed so that the woman's head is lower than her body, with the same pelvic tilting result (145).

Some form of lubrication will be applied to your abdomen; some doctors use the clear gel used for ultrasound scanning, some use talc (203), while others report (rather appealingly) using olive oil (139).

ECV, by virtue of its "external" definition does not generally require any vaginal examination. However, in cases where the baby's presenting part has deeply engaged, it has been suggested that two operators should be used, with one disengaging the presenting part from inside the vagina (203, 57). This is more likely to be necessary if your baby is an extended breech. If the presenting part cannot be disengaged it is likely that the attempt will fail (189). Although some authors routinely recommend two operators for ECV (22), it is more common for it to be carried out by only one person.

The doctor will start by lifting the baby up from the pelvis and then will locate the baby's head with one hand. By applying gentle pressure on the head and bottom, a "forward roll" can be attempted, at first turning the baby so that it is lying across your uterus and then continuing the half circle until the head is in your pelvis. If this is not successful, the doctor may attempt a "backward roll" – the same procedure in reverse (203). You may be asked to change position for this. Ideally the operator should wait for the uterus to become fully relaxed in between attempts (145). Overall the number of attempts is normally limited to three (145). Descriptions of how long it lasts vary enormously in the literature, with some suggesting that the procedure should last no longer than five minutes (203), and others lasting up to an hour (139).

If the version is successful, some authors suggest that you should stay lying flat for several minutes, presumably to give the baby a chance to settle in its new position (189). Other authors suggest that the baby's bottom should be gently pressed so as to direct the head more deeply into the pelvis (57). Presumably spending some time in a squatting position may also be beneficial. The proviso in the last chapter about ensuring that the baby is in a good position for a head down birth still holds – you do not want to be helping to engage a baby that is not well prepared for labour. If your baby is not well positioned it may be worth following some of the advice in Jean Sutton's book, *Understanding and Teaching Optimal Foetal Positioning* (279) (details in the Further Reading section at the back of this book).

The baby's heart rate should be checked at a minimum of every two minutes while ECV is taking place (189), and some doctors perform the entire procedure under ultrasound for monitoring both the baby and the progress of the procedure. Any significant abnormalities in the heart rate will lead to the procedure either being abandoned completely or stopped and re-started when the heart rate has returned to normal. Following completion of the procedure, whether or not it has been successful, the heart rate should be monitored to ensure normality. You should be kept under observation (or at least asked not to leave the hospital) for about half an hour in normal circumstances. If there are any abnormalities in the heart rate (which generally occur in approximately 1% of babies undergoing ECV (145)) this normally leads to further monitoring until normality has been regained. In rare circumstances you may have to proceed to an emergency caesarean.

In the days and weeks after the procedure, you should make sure you are paying attention to your baby's patterns of movements so that any reduction of these is picked up quickly and reported to your doctor, midwife or labour ward. Difficulties after ECV are rare and are discussed in more detail later in this chapter at "drawbacks and risks".

HOW DOES ECV FEEL?

This is a controversial area, with most of the literature describing ECV as causing no more than discomfort. Indeed, some doctors describe pain as a sign that something is wrong and suggest that the procedure should be stopped and restarted more gently once the pain has eased (129). The Midirs informed choice leaflet for women (see Further Reading section) states: "ECV can be uncomfortable but not painful", though it does add: "so far there haven't been any studies of what women think about it" (193). However, some of the accounts I have come across seem to have found the procedure painful. Emma described her experience thus:

It was the kind of pain you had to breathe through. Not sharp "something's wrong" pain, just hard work pain. It also made me sweat profusely and feel quite sick. I was exhausted afterwards. I remember thinking it was good preparation for labour as maybe my contractions would feel like this. A mother I knew told me it couldn't be anything like as bad as labour and that I was in for a shock when the birth started. I was right though, and in a way ECV was worse because it lasted longer than each contraction.

A published account of ECV went further:

I felt like I'd been punched in the ribs, stretched like leather. My attention focussed totally on my breath, which was forcing itself in and out with such intensity that I couldn't keep up with it. (234)

I have spoken to many midwives who suggest that pain is a sign of poor technique and not a necessary part of the procedure. However, knowing it may hurt should not necessarily put you off ECV (and should also not stop you from keeping your doctor or midwife informed about how you are feeling throughout the procedure). I wonder if some women have been through more anxiety during the procedure than they needed to because they have not been warned about how they may feel.

Despite the possible pain many women feel it is worth it. Clearly ECV is a boon when it is successful: "The baby was down! After months of dilemma, we could birth our child at home" (234).

Even when unsuccessful, some people may feel it helps them to focus on the birth and gives them a sense that they have done everything they can. Emma concluded "It didn't work but at least we tried. I wasn't left thinking 'If only we'd had a go' or 'What if....' I knew my baby was pretty settled where he was and we just had to plan for the birth."

Occasionally the procedure can be an emotional one. One woman, whose ECV was successful, said (after the procedure was over): "I started sobbing, and tears were everywhere" (234). It is likely that you may feel tired after the procedure so it is probably best not to schedule anything too hectic for the rest of your day. Where possible you may well want your partner to be with you (particularly because of the risk, albeit small, of triggering labour or needing a caesarean section).

THE HISTORY OF ECV

ECV has been described in medical literature since the writings of Hippocrates (209). Aristotle stated that authors of his time advised midwives confronted with breech presentations to place the head so that it presents at birth (189). There is evidence that it was practised throughout the European middle ages (145) and in the 1500s Ambroise Pare, surgeon to the King of France, pioneered the techniques of version and extraction (57). At that time, internal version was also used in cases of transverse lie. The birth attendant inserted a hand into the uterus, grasped the baby by its feet, turned it and then pulled it out, still holding the feet.

The first detailed written description of the procedure appeared in 1807 by Wigand who practised ECV during labour between contractions (189). Hubert wrote in 1843 of "correcting 'vicious' presentations of the fetus by external manipulations" (275). During the nineteenth century, a combined version using an internal and an external hand emerged. Some of these could only be used in late labour as they required a large degree of cervical dilation. Busch, for example, recommended inserting the hand inside the uterus and seizing the head to turn it round, while Wright and d'Outrepont suggested grasping the shoulder. Hall and Braxton Hicks (of the pre-labour contractions fame) refined the technique so that only two fingers were inserted into the uterus to effect the version, enabling the procedure to be carried out much earlier in labour. This method, known as "bipolar version" was thought to be one of the most important contributions to obstetrics in the nineteenth century (57).

Vartan wrote in 1940 that ECV simply mimicked the natural physiological procedure occurring in many women at 32–33 weeks of pregnancy (303). By the late 1930s and early 1940s a series of large population studies on as many as 1105 women in one study led Stevenson to conclude in 1951 that the "risk to the mother or baby from ECV is far less than the risk of delivery" (275). ECV remained popular in the 1960s and early 1970s, and there were further large studies showing the success of the technique (233). Routine use of ECV was common up to the 1970s, often being carried out in ante-natal clinics (189).

The three factors which led to a significant decline in the practice of ECV were:

1. questions over the effectiveness of the procedure following frequent observations of babies turning back to being breech after a successful ECV
2. related to (1), questions over any improvement over the spontaneous turning rate (i.e., ECV was turning babies who would have turned anyway)
3. concerns over the safety of the procedure for the baby, following reports of death rates attributable to the procedure being as high as 1.6% (32) and complications as high as 4.4% (33).

Interestingly the death rate argument was initially not seen as a problem because it was lower than the death rate occurring during breech birth. As the death rates for breech babies fell, the relative risks of ECV started to seem greater, leading one author to write in 1975 that "ECV can only do positive harm" and to conclude that "a routine policy of ECV cannot be justified" (33). However, in the same year a study was published examining the effects of carrying out ECV at term (i.e. 36 weeks or more) (247). Up to this time, ECV was generally carried out much earlier in pregnancy, around 32 weeks. Carrying out ECV at term had the triple advantage of reducing the number of unnecessary ECV attempts on babies who would have turned anyway if left to their own devices, avoiding the hazards of prematurity if the baby needed to be born immediately after the procedure as a result of fetal distress, and giving more opportunity for any possible contraindications to the procedure to make themselves evident. This study also contains one of the early reports of routine monitoring using cardiotocography following ECV attempts. Hughes stated in 1998 that "the improved ability to assess the welfare of the fetus has decreased the risk of the procedure, which is now less than that of either a vaginal or abdominal breech delivery" (139).

This chequered history has left considerable diversity of opinion about ECV as expressed by MacArthur (233): "There are those who enthusiastically recommend it, others who violently oppose it, and still others who express a rather elegant distaste for it." Despite further developments in the research and national policies recommending the routine provision of ECV, this diversity amongst clinicians persists today.

THE CURRENT STATUS OF ECV

To date there have been six randomised controlled trials of ECV (35, 134, 181, 298, 299, 301) which were brought together in a meta-analysis by Hofmeyr in 1998. A meta-analysis pools the results of studies which all meet certain methodological criteria, and can thus base its conclusions on a much larger sample than any single study is able to. Hofmeyr concluded that there is a significant reduction in the risk of a caesarean section for women undergoing ECV without any increased risk to the baby (135). Based on a similar meta-analysis in 1993, the Royal College of Obstetricians and Gynaecologists (RCOG) of Great Britain stated that "all women with an uncomplicated breech pregnancy at term should be offered ECV" (236). They asked obstetricians to set this as a standard to be evaluated in all units in the UK. In addition it was stated "a skilled service should be available and offered", placing consultants under some obligation to ensure that ECV is offered by a doctor with experience of the technique. Similarly, the American College of Obstetricians and Gynaecologists (ACOG) concluded in a review of ECV in 1997 that "all women with near term breech presentations should be offered a version attempt" (10). Myerscough (203) stated in 1998: "After adequate randomised trials, ECV is now clearly re-established as part of the proper management of breech presentation."

CONTRAINDICATIONS

Contraindications are factors which make the application of a technique or intervention inadvisable. They can be divided into absolute and relative. Absolute contraindications are sufficient to rule out the option of ECV. Relative contraindications would be considered as possible deterrents to the procedure but would need to be considered on an "individualised care" basis (145).

There is a good general consensus about factors which make women absolutely unsuitable for ECV due to an increase in the risk associated with the procedure. The presence of any one of the characteristics described in Table 5.1 is sufficient to rule out the option of ECV.

Table 5.1   List of absolute contraindications to ECV

Multiple pregnancy
Significant third trimester bleeding
Placenta praevia
Premature rupture of the fetal membranes
Severe pre-eclampsia
Hyperextended fetal head
Caesarean section necessary for other reasons

Pre-eclampsia and bleeding are only considered a relative contraindication by Johanson (145). The ACOG review listed the contraindications shown in Table 5.2 in addition as reasons not to offer ECV, though it did not differentiate between absolute and relative contraindications (10).

Table 5.2   ACOG list of additional contraindications

Evidence of uteroplacental insufficiency
Suspected intrauterine growth restriction
Amniotic fluid abnormalities
Uterine malformation
Maternal cardiac disease
Pregnancy induced hypertension
Uncontrolled hypertension
A nonreassuring fetal monitoring pattern
Major fetal abnormality

McParland and Farine (189) also include on their list of relative contraindications previous caesarean section, diabetes and obesity. However, they go on to point out that in the case of gestational diabetes, mild hypertension and a previous caesarean scar there have been recent reports that ECV can in fact be performed safely. In the case of previous caesarean section, Flamm et al. (101) found a relatively high success rate of 82% in 56 women who had had one or more caesarean sections with no complications arising from the procedure.[1] Another study found that ECV was safe and effective in 38 women with a previous caesarean section (80). The reason for this appearing as a contraindication for ECV relates to concerns about the rupture of the uterine scar during the procedure. However, in the same way that this concern was seen as a contraindication to vaginal birth after caesarean and has now been successfully challenged in much of the UK at least (109, 287), it seems that ECV may now become increasingly available to women with previous caesarean section. The ACOG are somewhat cautious about their conclusions on this saying that larger trials are needed to determine the risk of uterine rupture. Johanson (145) differentiates between a classical caesarean section (a vertical scar), which he rates as an absolute contraindication, along with other previous uterine surgery, and a lower segment caesarean section (the more common "bikini line" scar) which he considers a relative contraindication. Recent research appears to suggest that the layers of suturing or stitches may also have a key role to play in the risk of uterine rupture. One layer of suturing appears to be associated with higher levels of rupture than two layers of suturing (69).

The ACOG's contraindications are based on "a commonsense approach" rather than research evidence (110). As such they may tend to veer on the side of caution. The ACOG's placing of cardiac disease on its original list leaves one wondering whether an estimation of the relative risks of ECV and for example caesarean section have been undertaken. It seems possible that an ECV attempt, albeit with careful monitoring of the woman with heart disease as well as her baby, may be

---

1. The key here is the nature of the uterine incision, which may not correlate with the scar on the skin. It is possible to have a vertical uterine incision and a bikini line scar (108).

worthwhile. It is interesting that maternal cardiac disease does not appear on some other lists of contraindications to ECV (145, 189, 203).

The ACOG's contraindications also have a joint function, designed to "minimize the risks of an adverse outcome and to maximize the chances for success". The problem with this, which is a common feature in lists of contraindications for ECV, is that criteria which make the procedure more risky are combined with features which may not be unsafe but make the procedure more likely to fail. While these two factors may both be relevant, particularly for a busy doctor, they are important to differentiate for women who would obviously want to avoid putting their baby at risk but may be keen to try ECV even if the chances of success are low. Perhaps the least risky on the ACOG list is amniotic fluid abnormalities. Some studies have shown that reduced amniotic fluid volume is associated with less success (131, 137, 260) while others have failed to show such a relationship (209). Similarly obesity has been associated with lower success rates in one study (35), whereas many others did not find it to be a significant predictor of success (131, 209, 260, 282). If you are a woman who wants ECV, particularly if you have other characteristics that make ECV more likely to succeed such as previous children or a flexed breech, you should not be denied the opportunity on the basis of reduced fluid volume or obesity. Factors influencing the success of ECV are discussed in Chapter 6 in more detail.

Only one paper that I came across included "patient reluctance/refusal" as an absolute contraindication (145). Guy Thorpe-Beeston commented that "Some women have a gut feeling that they don't feel comfortable trying to turn the baby" (293). Jean Robinson from the Association for Improvements in Maternity Services points out that some women feel very protective about their babies by this stage in pregnancy and are reluctant to expose them to ECV, believing that it may cause their babies pain or trauma (242). Your view of ECV is also influenced by your view of why the baby is breech in the first place. If you believe it is lying breech because it is comfortable that way, or is somehow meant to be that way, ECV is likely to seem more disruptive and intrusive. Just as you have a right to ask for ECV, you equally have a right to turn it down if it does not feel like the right decision for you.

SUCCESS RATES

Success rates for ECV vary between 25% (131) and 90% (322) with one report from a doctor very experienced in the technique claiming a 90.9% success rate (233). The range of factors likely to account for this variation are explored in depth in the next chapter.

DRAWBACKS AND RISKS OF ECV

It is now routinely stated in publications for women (193) and professionals that ECV is safe. However, "safe" implies a risk free procedure which is not, strictly speaking, the case. It is true that there are some studies that report no serious adverse outcomes at all (257, 139). Those that do report problems often report fetal distress which is transitory and resolves swiftly (129, 139, 209, 166). For example, Healey et al. reported six abnormal CTGs (heart rate patterns) during or after ECV in their sample of 89 women. All of these returned to normal within two hours and there were no further problems reported (129).

However, there are reports of very occasional fetal deaths in the literature. Michel Odent has also suggested that accidents may occur that do not appear in the literature. Healey et al. (129) reported one death in their study two days after an unsuccessful attempt at ECV. There had been a small haemorrhage and an episode of hypoxia, although all of the monitoring following ECV had been normal. The authors simply state "No cause was found for the hypoxia" but do not rule out the possible role of ECV in causing it.

One study entitled "Fetal demise following ECV" reports a case of a healthy woman whose ECV was successful with normal monitoring before and after the procedure (188). However, three days later she re-presented with a loss of fetal movements and the baby was found to have died. At birth the baby was found to have a tight knot in its umbilical cord. The authors state that although the overall risk of ECV is small, for their patient "the risk is absolute" and conclude that ECV poses a "definite and sometimes unpreventable risk of cord accident". Although these authors report the use of all the normal monitoring, it is unclear the extent to which they used ultrasound during the procedure. Whether this would have detected the cord knot is uncertain. Donald Gibb stated that although a radiographer with skill and obstetric experience would be able to detect the location of the cord, the average radiographer is unlikely to be able to do so (115). This raises the question of the level of skill which should be demanded for ECV ultrasound and whether current practice is satisfactory.

One extremely rare complication, to the point of being unheard of by many practitioners, is found in a paper entitled "Uterine rotation following attempted ECV" (56). The woman in this case study was found to have a baby in transverse lie (lying across her uterus) at 36 weeks of pregnancy and was offered ECV. After four unsuccessful attempts a caesarean section was scheduled. During the section it was observed that the uterus had rotated. The baby was fine.

Reports of babies dying doubtless make chilling reading for any pregnant woman considering ECV and as with many aspects of this book I have debated its inclusion, knowing the emotional impact it could have. However, it is important for you to have all the information so that you can make an informed choice. Ultimately the deaths and complications reported here could be explained by problems of technique or monitoring failures in the study concerned. The risks are very small when seen in the context of the large body of research which supports its use, and the representative bodies of midwives, obstetricians and gynaecologists in many countries support the practice of ECV. McParland and Farine conclude: "Although the risks [of ECV] to the fetus are not negligible, performing ECV at term with appropriate facilities appears to be a proven and effective form of care" (189). The risks should also be seen in the context of the other risks which may arise from giving birth to a breech as opposed to a head down baby. We know that there are higher risks to both mother and baby from having a caesarean section (see Chapter 12) as opposed to a head down vaginal birth. Assessing the risks or otherwise of a vaginal breech birth is complicated by those who argue that any higher risk is caused by mismanagement of the process rather than any factor inherent in vaginal breech birth itself. However, it is important that you consider the risks of ECV in relation to any potential risks of the mode of delivery you are planning. One important message to take from this information is that ECV is not a procedure to be taken lightly and that it seems highly inadvisable to do it away from a hospital, as does occasionally still happen (234).

One drawback which does not compromise your baby's health directly but may have an impact if you are considering attempting a vaginal birth is the possibility that a baby with its bottom presenting at the cervix could be shifted so that its feet present at the cervix. A report of such an occurrence appears in Naomi Wolf's book *Misconceptions* (318). Unfortunately it is not clear whether the baby had its legs extended initially or was a complete breech with legs flexed (the latter would be more likely). You should discuss this possibility first with whoever is likely to be with you in labour. Some professionals are comfortable with footling breech births, but others would consider this to be a contraindication to a vaginal breech birth. This possibility, though remote, may affect your decision about whether to have ECV. If you are planning a caesarean this is not a concern.

One final drawback of ECV, though it is a drawback relevant to services and opportunities for the future, rather than individual women, is that the more it is practised successfully, the less opportunity there is for vaginal breech birth expertise to be developed and maintained (139). In itself this does not seem to be a good reason not to have ECV, but is an unwanted spin-off from the growing prevalence of this intervention.

CURRENT PRACTICE OF ECV

In spite of the advice from the Royal College that ECV should be universally offered to all women with uncomplicated term pregnancy, results from a study conducted in 1995 indicate that only 48% of obstetricians perform ECV (63). This percentage increases to 55% when those who refer women to a colleague for the procedure are included. This means that 45% of obstetricians neither perform ECV nor offer women in their care the opportunity to have ECV performed by a colleague. In fact, this is likely to be an underestimate as the response rate to the questionnaire was 78%. Coltart et al. point out that this could bias the results towards those who are practising ECV (i.e., those not performing ECV would be less likely to return the questionnaire), suggesting that the real percentage of obstetricians not offering ECV could be higher still (63).

Interestingly, there was significant national variation in ECV practice, with by far the lowest percentages of ECV occurring in England and Wales. Table 5.3 shows the range in ECV and how this impacts upon breech births and caesarean sections.

As the figures in Table 5.3 suggest, rather unsurprisingly, there is a significant inverse relationship between the amount of ECV performed and both the number of breech births and caesarean sections performed for breech. Coltart et al. estimate that if ECV was universally applied, 6600 breech births could be prevented each year (63). With a caesarean section rate for breech of 70% in 1993 (12) this translates into 4600 preventable caesareans.

Table 5.3   Prevalence of ECV, breech birth and caesarean section for breech

Area	No. of consultants performing ECV or referring on (% of total)	Breech birth (cs+vb*) (% of all births)	Caesarean section for breech (% of all births)
England	361 (50%)	21,038 (3.56%)	14,546 (2.46%)
Scotland	79 (77%)	1490 (2.67%)	1039 (1.86%)
Wales	24 (49%)	1267 (3.68%)	869 (2.52%)
Northern Ireland	37 (82%)	546 (2.19%)	307 (1.23%)
Republic of Ireland	39 (74%)	1297 (3.0%)	843 (1.95%)

*These figures are for all breech births, vaginal and caesarean.

Source: Coltart, T., et al. External Cephalic Version. *British Journal of Obstetrics and Gynaecology* 104 (1997): 544–7. Reprinted with permission from Elsevier Science.

The situation in America is likely to be similar. Spelliscy-Gifford and colleagues commented in 1995 (270) that ECV in America did not appear to be widespread because the overall rates of breech birth had not reduced. Some American researchers have attempted to quantify the financial cost of failing to offer ECV (187, 270) and found that it is considerable. One study (187) estimated that each successful version saved $2462 in 1996 (with a relatively low success rate of 48%). They suggested that if they improved their success rate to 62% by targeting their ECV attempts to those women more likely to succeed their institution would save $34,000 per 100 patients. They also suggest that using the results of another study suggesting that routine use of cephalic version (270) could result in a 1% reduction in the US caesarean rate nationally, at least $30 million per year could be saved. These savings are likely to be an underestimate as they only include the immediate costs of the method of delivery itself and do not include any costs arising from problems in the mother or baby after the birth. Since maternal morbidity and extended hospital stay following caesarean section is well documented, the real cost of not offering ECV is likely to be significantly higher.

The multi-centre trial indicated that nearly 80% of participants had not had an attempt at ECV (127), an alarmingly high figure.

What this research does not convey, of course, is the real emotional costs of breech birth in the current obstetric climate, both the apprehension before and dealing with the aftermath of any birth related problems for mother or baby. The fact that some of this is preventable by the routine offering of ECV is simply inexcusable.

WHY YOU MIGHT NOT BE OFFERED ECV

As observed earlier, many consultants remain "violently opposed" to ECV (189) and it is not unusual for women who ask about ECV to be told by midwives and doctors that ECV is a dangerous and outmoded procedure.

The prejudice against the technique is even reported in the literature. Hughes reports that one of his consultant colleagues at a hospital in Plymouth "would not allow his patients to be referred for ECV" (139). Maggie Banks (17) reports an anecdote of a "bright young registrar presenting a teaching session on breech, following which one consultant obstetrician commented that 'ECV was now outdated with [the use of] caesarean section [for breech]'. When the registrar drew attention to the long ago reported value of ECV at term...he was met with a 'watch it boy!'"

Even where ECV is "offered", the manner of its offering can affect the uptake of the offer as Johanson (145) points out: "It can be difficult for professionals to conceal their own innate prejudices or beliefs, and 'negative vibes' are important influences." Despite the RCOG guidelines being published in 1993 and subsequent leaflets summarising these and the research on ECV for professionals being issued (193), it seems that this information is yet to permeate many pockets of the NHS.

The problem is likely to be to a great extent one of training. Coltart points out that in the past, training on ECV has only happened in the workplace and is thus entirely dependent on whether a particular consultant offers it. With such variation in practice, he comments "it would only have been by chance that obstetric training would have included learning how to perform ECV" (63). Spelliscy-Gifford et al. (270) make a similar point about American obstetricians and suggest that residency training (i.e., training on placement rather than in medical school) is insufficient. They comment that "Practitioners may feel more comfortable performing caesareans, even though it is a more complex procedure."

McParland and Farine suggest a practical approach to solving the training obstacle (189). They point out that the technique can be learned quickly and that witnessing a few ECVs should be sufficient to prepare doctors to attempt several versions under supervision. Since only one doctor per hospital needs to be trained to set up an ECV clinic (passing on their expertise as required), training could be carried out with only a few visits to another hospital's ECV clinic. Three or four half days of training is a minimal time outlay when compared to the benefits of starting an ECV clinic. Hughes reports that in his study the learning curves to achieve an acceptable success rate were relatively short, occurring consistently after 15 version attempts (139).

Some professionals may remain opposed to ECV despite their awareness of current research. This seems a legitimate position so long as they explain to their patients why they do not agree with ECV and provide the option of ECV with a colleague (or at least explain how women can gain access to ECV if they wish to).

Some hospitals will claim practical difficulties with offering ECV. As discussed earlier, it is now thought to be safest to carry out ECV with access to an operating theatre so that the doctor can proceed to an emergency caesarean section in the unlikely event of this being necessary. In theory this requires the consultant offering ECV to have access to theatre time during ECV clinics. This has led one hospital to claim, when challenged for not offering ECV, "As we do not have external version lists [operating theatre time] at hospital x, we are not able to offer this service" (199). In fact, this seems little more than dodging the issue. Routine practice of ECV is unlikely to lead to significant numbers of emergency caesareans.

In the same way that any emergency caesarean is fitted in, prioritising the urgency of existing patients, it is difficult to understand how this cannot be arranged for ECV. Hughes, in his 1998 review of the value of ECV, says that ECV clinics can be undertaken at a time when staffing levels make it easier to cope with an emergency caesarean section in the unlikely event of the need arising (139).

However, although this particular objection is relatively straightforward to argue away, it may well be a smokescreen for a general lack of interest in, enthusiasm for or experience of ECV, and you may find yourself needing to transfer to a different hospital.

WHAT TO DO IF YOU ARE NOT OFFERED ECV AND YOU WANT IT

In order to help you feel stronger in your request for ECV you may want to obtain a copy of the Midirs leaflet on breech birth (193) which you can ask your midwife for. If your midwife is not able to provide you with one then you could try contacting Midirs directly (for contact details see the useful contacts section at the back of this book). If you are not offered ECV at 36–37 weeks then ask your doctor if there is any reason why you should not have ECV (see "Contraindications" above). If there is not, ask if there is anyone at your hospital with experience of ECV. If the answer is in the negative, ask if you can be referred to another hospital for the procedure. Although you may not be considering transferring hospitals for the birth if your baby remains breech (see Chapter 13), there is no reason why you cannot be transferred to another consultant or hospital for this procedure alone and return to your hospital for the birth. It is analogous to a patient requiring a scan using a piece of equipment which one hospital does not possess. It would be routine for them to be referred to another hospital for the scan and then sent back for the rest of their medical care. Another example is the use of special care baby units which are not present at every maternity unit.

If you do not make progress with your consultant, you should discuss the issue with your GP. Because you are still under the care of your consultant, your GP may be reluctant to make a referral to another consultant, feeling that this referral should come from your consultant. However, if you explain that you have tried this route, your GP should be willing to either make a referral him/herself or discuss it with the consultant on your behalf. The late Dr Richard Johanson stated that "It is the GP's responsibility to seek out a consultant who practices ECV for his patients" and concluded his article by urging: "If ECV is not offered at your local hospital, try further afield!" (145).

If you have a supportive midwife she may be able to help, perhaps in playing an advocate role for you with your consultant, or by discussing the situation with your GP, or by finding out about which hospitals locally offer ECV. However, she does not have the power to refer you elsewhere.

Ideally, if ECV is not offered by your hospital, someone involved in your care should know or be able to find out somewhere that does. However, if this support is not forthcoming, you may need to do some of the research yourself. Once you have found out which other hospitals in your area have maternity units, it is probably easiest to telephone and ask to speak to the Director of Midwifery services, or at least a senior midwife to find out whether ECV is offered, and if so by which doctors. They are likely to be busy people and you may need to keep trying in order to get hold of them. However, your conversation should only need to be brief and they should not mind giving you the time.

You may not have many options of different hospitals open to you, particularly if you don't live in or near a big city. If you are struggling to find a hospital that offers ECV, or the only one you can find involves significant travel you may decide to reconsider your decision to try ECV. In doing so you may want to think about the factors influencing the outcome of ECV described in the next chapter. If you have several characteristics that suggest ECV is more likely to be successful, it may be more worth your while seeking ECV than if you do not.

SUMMARY

Despite a chequered history, ECV is now generally thought to be a safe and effective procedure for turning breech babies. It is offered on an out-patient basis after 37 weeks. It may hurt. There are factors which may make ECV inappropriate in particular cases (contraindications), including a hyperextended fetal head, placenta praevia, and severe pre-eclampsia. If you need a caesarean for reasons other than your baby being breech, ECV is not appropriate. The RCOG recommends that all women with a breech baby should be offered ECV. However, a survey published in 1995 suggested that on average only 55% of consultants were offering or referring women on for ECV. If you are not, and want to, you can ask to be referred elsewhere. If you do not wish to have ECV, you do not have to.

6
Factors Influencing the Success of External Cephalic Version (ECV)

INTRODUCTION

Success rates for ECV vary widely. This chapter explores factors which may account for this variation and interventions which may make ECV more likely to succeed. Please note that this chapter may include more information than you want or need about ECV. Feel free to ignore it completely or dip into it for reference only. The interventions described to try to improve the success of ECV include the use of medication (tocolysis), repetition, carrying out ECV with an epidural in place and/or after labour has started and carrying out ECV earlier than recommended. Research relating to these various interventions is described along with some indication as to whether your doctor is likely to be willing to use such an intervention.

SUCCESS RATES AND FACTORS INFLUENCING SUCCESS

Success rates for ECV vary between 25% (131) and 90% (322) – an unusual degree of variation for any medical intervention. There are likely to be several reasons for this variation. Different exclusion criteria certainly account for some of the variability in outcome. The varying proportion of women with no previous children is likely to contribute as is the ethnic background of the sample (see below). It is also possible that there are also considerable variations in different doctors' skill levels.

The factor most reliably associated with successful ECV is the number of previous pregnancies the woman has had (parity). This is unsurprising as this is also the factor most strongly associated with spontaneous turning. The greater space in the uterus and greater flexibility of the abdominal walls of the woman who has had previous pregnancies make turning much easier. Success rates for women with no previous children can be as low as 39% (131) while those for women with previous children can be as high as 80% (131).

It is also generally accepted that non-engagement is a good predictor of successful ECV. This is thought to account for higher success rates of ECV in women of African descent. One study which found a 90% success rate in Africa suggested that this was due to a difference in the shape of the pelvis, meaning that babies were less likely to engage (322). Transverse lie is also thought to be a good predictor of success, sometimes achieving success rates of 100% (131).

It is also generally thought that flexed fetal legs make ECV easier, something that would also be expected from the association between flexed fetal legs and spontaneous turning (314). Hellstrom et al. (131) provide an interesting breakdown of their sample of the baby's position and the outcome of ECV shown in Table 6.1. The terminology used in the table, which is discussed in detail in Chapter 1, is somewhat confusing. The important comparison is between flexed and extended breech.

Table 6.1   Baby's position and outcome of ECV

Baby's position	Number of babies	Number of successful ECV	% success
Extended legs	163	74	45% *
No prev. preg.		31	31%
One+ prev. preg.		43	67%
Incomplete flexed breech:			
Singleton footling breech	41	24	59%
Double footling breech	66	53	80%**
Complete flexed breech:			
Double foot	12	7	58%
Transverse lie	11	11	100%***

* Significantly lower than the rest of the sample combined.
** Significantly higher than the rest of the sample combined.
*** Group too small to perform statistical significance, though results suggest strong relationship between transverse lie and success of ECV.

Source: Hellstrom, A.C., et al. When does external cephalic version succeed? Reprinted with permission from *Acta Obstetricia et Gynecologica Scandinavica* 69 (1990): 281–5.

Another study found even greater success with flexed breeches (complete only), turning 96% as opposed to 65% with extended breeches (98). However, one study found the opposite to this, with higher success rates with extended breeches (71%) than with flexed breeches (complete – 53%; incomplete – 30%) (83).

One study found that a difficulty in feeling the baby's head, due to its being hidden under an area in the upper part of the uterus, was associated with lower success rates (166). A similar factor related to positioning is lower success being associated with babies whose backs are posterior. This is because only the soft parts of the baby's body are accessible to the ECV operator which makes manipulation more difficult (98, 104).

Other factors related to the outcome of ECV have been dogged by inconsistent findings. As already discussed in the previous chapter, insufficient amniotic fluid is widely believed to make ECV more difficult, to the point that it is used as a contraindication by some, and yet some studies fail to find an association between fluid volume and ECV success. As also mentioned in the previous chapter, obesity is believed by some to be a contraindication but the relationship between obesity and low success rates has not been demonstrated consistently. In relation to the size of the baby, some studies have found that babies weighing over 4000g are more difficult to turn (240) whereas others failed to find such a link between success and size (98, 184). Some studies report an association between the location of the placenta and ECV outcome (137, 209, 35, 38, 98) while others do not (83, 131,

260). These associations are not straightforward, as some found anterior placental locations to correlate with failure (35, 209), while others found cornual implantations to relate to failure (98, 137) (see Chapter 2 for a description of different placental locations).

This uncertainty led Hellstrom et al. (131) to conclude that one "cannot easily predict cases in which ECV is bound to be unsuccessful", pointing out that even in the women with no previous children and babies with extended legs they achieved a success rate of 31%. In light of this they suggest that ECV must always be worth a try where there are no clear contraindications.

One interesting study by Newman et al. in 1993 identified a range of factors associated with ECV success in a group of 286 women (209). They used this information to develop a scoring system (see Table 6.2 below) which they then applied to a new group of 286 women. They found that women scoring less than or equal to 2 on a 0–10 scale had no successful versions, whereas all women with a score of 9 or 10 had successful versions. Table 6.2 shows the scoring system they used with terms explained briefly. The scoring system would require the help of your midwife or obstetrician on some of the items.

Table 6.2   Newman et al.'s scoring system for estimating the likelihood of successful ECV (209)

Score	0	1	2
Characteristic			
Parity*	0	1	>2
Dilatation of cervix	>3cm	1–2cm	0cm
Estimated weight	<2500g	2500–3500g	>3500g
Placenta	anterior	posterior	lateral/fundal
Station**	>–1	–2	<–3

* Number of previous pregnancies
** Station is a measure of engagement with –3 being higher in the uterus than –1

Source: Newman, R.B. et al., Predicting the success of external cephalic version. *American Journal of Obstetrics and Gynecology* (1993): 245–9.

The ACOG review cautions that these results have not been validated by multiple studies and state that no single scoring system has been found to have complete accuracy (10). They suggest that studies such as this one can be used to provide women with the information they need to make informed consent. In the discussion at the end of the last chapter on accessing ECV when it is not provided at your local hospital, I have suggested that when ECV is difficult to organise, you may decide it is not worth the hassle if the likelihood of success looks as if it will be low. This scoring system may help with making that decision.

INTERVENTIONS AIMED AT IMPROVING THE SUCCESS OF ECV

What follows is a review of variations or additions to the standard technique of ECV that may improve success rates. Some may be offered to you routinely, others may be straightforward to request, while others may be more difficult to access. I have tried to present the interventions according to a rough order of accessibility. The last intervention on the list, transabdominal amnioinfusion is still in the stages of early research and it is highly unlikely that you will be able to access it.

Training women to identify reversion to breech following successful ECV

There is only one study (270) that deals with this issue, referred to earlier in the section on "how can you tell your baby has turned?" in Chapter 4. The context for this unusual decision to give women this degree of involvement in their care was an African obstetric service with scarce obstetrical resources and poor outcomes from breech birth. The authors wanted to see if they could increase the efficacy of ECV still further by training women who had had successful versions to assess their baby's position, with a view to re-presenting to the obstetrician in the event of a suspected reversion to breech.

The intervention was successful, in terms of significantly more repeat versions being carried out in the intervention group, translating into significantly more head down births compared to a control group. Of the 12 women in the intervention group returning with suspected reversion to breech 10 were right, leading the authors to comment that women's ability to detect reversion to breech was "surprisingly good". The main issue affecting the applicability of this study to other women (apart from the oft found Western medical resistance to women's involvement in their care) is the higher frequency of spontaneous reversion to breech in African women. It could therefore be argued that it is less cost effective to train Caucasian women than African women. However, comparing the cost of a caesarean section, or even a vaginal delivery with all the medical personnel normally required for a breech birth to the minimal cost of a brief training session on assessment of fetal lie, it would appear to still make good financial sense even if it prevented only 1 breech birth in 50–100. There are also the considerable psychological benefits of involving women more in their care, and enabling women to be more confident in using alternative approaches to turning.

If you are interested in learning to identify your baby's position, ask your midwife to show you how.

Tocolysis (medication) and ECV

Tocolysis refers to the use of medication to relax the muscles of the uterus. Many of the published studies use tocolysis routinely as an adjunct to ECV (131, 38, 165, 121, 260, 86, 201, 277, 295, 28, 181). The most commonly used tocolytic medication is ritodrine, but one study found another agent, hexoprenaline, to be associated with higher success rates (278). Another drug in the same group, terbutaline may also be used. These drugs are all classed as "myometrial relaxants" – in essence their action relaxes the muscles of the uterus. They are most commonly used to try to inhibit contractions in premature labour. Side effects can include nausea, vomiting, flushing, sweating, tremors, palpitations, chest pain or tightness and hypotension (low blood pressure). It is recommended that where low blood pressure may be a problem, the woman lies on her left side where possible. Although the list is an alarming one, lists of side effects generally are, even for drugs which many of us may use regularly (such as paracetamol or aspirin). The exposure to the drug during ECV is also far briefer than exposure when premature labour is being treated, when treatment is recommended for up to 48 hours. These drugs are not thought to harm your baby.

There have been five randomised controlled trials to date on the use of tocolysis. Two of these showed no benefit of tocolysis (282, 240) and one showed benefit of hexoprenaline but not ritodrine (278). The remaining two showed advantages of tocolysis with women with no previous pregnancies (54, 185) and one of these showed that this effect was most apparent when the technique of ECV was being learned by the operator (54). One study using tocolysis found a reduced incidence of fetal bradycardia (an abnormally slow heart rate) during the procedure and a more rapid completion of ECV (278).

The ACOG review concludes that routine use of a tocolytic may not be justified in women who have had one or more previous pregnancies when the chances of success without tocolysis are already high. Myerscough states that tocolysis is "a valuable aid, especially for the learner, but not an absolute prerequisite" (203). There is evidence that "learners" may need extra help. One study found that although the learning curve was relatively quick and no further gains were made after the first 20 patients, success rates increased from an initial 45% to 60% (285). So if you are having ECV with a relatively inexperienced doctor you have good reason to ask to be transferred to someone more experienced, or to ask for tocolysis to be used.

Some authors have suggested that the use of a tocolysis should depend on the results of the initial examination of the patient (189). McParland and Farine state: "If the uterus is relaxed, this seems unnecessary." It has also been cautioned that tocolytics will only relax the walls of the uterus, and that tension in the abdominal muscles can be equally problematic for the procedure (115). Their effectiveness may therefore be limited.

Although there are no reported side effects of ritodrine thought to be harmful to the baby, the woman's blood pressure should be checked regularly. In rare cases can lead to fainting and collapse (145). If you are concerned about the use of medication in your pregnancy and your doctor is suggesting using tocolysis, you can ask to have an attempt at ECV without tocolysis. Equally if you are not being offered tocolysis and would like to try it, ask if this can be done. Of all the procedures described in this section, tocolysis is the most researched and should be the easiest "add-on" to straight ECV to access.

Repetition

Policy statements are frequently somewhat vague regarding repeat attempts following unsuccessful ECV, often suggesting that repetition is an option but not giving any clear basis on which the decision to repeat is made.

Dr Ranney, in a delightful paper written in 1973 entitled "The gentle art of ECV", describes repeated attempts at ECV as being an integral part of his practice (233). He believes this contributes to the right attitude towards ECV: "This is no place for a hasty or domineering approach which is futile and possibly dangerous...If not today, then probably at the next office visit."

He reported that of the 25 women whose babies did not turn at the first ECV attempt, but did eventually, 16 turned on the second attempt, 5 turned on the third attempt, 1 on the fourth and 3 on the fifth. He also reported one case of an initially successful version which turned back to being breech which took eight further attempts at ECV before it stayed head down. The important proviso to bear in mind when interpreting these results is that Ranney starts ECV between 30 and 34 weeks so many of his repeat turns would be occurring earlier than 36 weeks.

Interestingly he found that in 27 of his patients whose initial attempt at ECV had failed, a spontaneous version occurred. He suggests that this may be due to the ECV attempt realigning the baby's positions to make it easier to turn (though of course it may simply be the babies who would have turned on their own anyway, particularly given his practice of ECV early in pregnancy).

Nevertheless, Ranney's success rate of 90.9% is impressive, and suggests that investing more time in ECV, rather than giving up after one failed attempt, may be worthwhile.

Fetal acoustic stimulation

Fetal acoustic stimulation involves the application of a noise to the abdomen which elicits a "startle response" from the baby (i.e., the baby "jumps"). The resulting movement and heart rate changes facilitate repositioning of the fetus using ECV. The use of fetal acoustic stimulation in obstetrics is expanding, with its use both ante-natally (to facilitate ultrasound and in ante-natal testing) and in labour (to evaluate fetal well-being). There have been no reported adverse outcomes, and in a large long-term follow-up study of children in whom fetal acoustic stimulation had been used before birth, no evidence of any hearing problems emerged (13).

Dr Johnson and colleagues published two studies in 1995 relating to the efficacy of the technique (146, 147) and found highly promising results. The technique involves applying the acoustic stimulation to the abdomen for one to three seconds. ECV is then attempted. In a well-designed controlled trial, an 86% success rate was found, which is at the upper end of the range of success rates for ECV. This high success rate may have been at least partly influenced by their exclusion of babies with engagement of the presenting part, and by their protocol of two attempts at ECV. Nevertheless, their results are encouraging and it seems possible that this may be offered as an adjunct to ECV increasingly in the future, though the fact that there have been no further reports of its use since 1995 may suggest that its use is not widespread.

Epidural anaesthesia and ECV

There has been concern about the use of epidural anaesthesia in ECV because of a fear that too much force might be used, leading to possible harm to mother or baby. Many authors describe using reports of maternal pain as an indication to stop the procedure immediately (129), a source of information clearly not available with a successful pain blocking epidural in place. However, early reports of the possible benefits of epidurals for the success rates of ECV in the US (42, 99) have led to increasing willingness to evaluate their role further.

There are two randomised controlled trials relating to the use of epidural anaesthesia and ECV. The first found a significantly higher success rate of 69% in women with epidurals, versus 32% without, in a sample of 69 women. The authors found no evidence of any harm to mother or baby (257). However the second found no benefit to epidural in a sample of 102 women (84).

The use of epidural anaesthesia is clearly a more costly adjunct to ECV than some of the others mentioned above. However, the authors of this study argue that the cost is more than offset by the shortened hospital stay when ECV is successful and caesareans are avoided. They also went on to perform a caesarean in those women for whom ECV was unsuccessful (and where elective caesarean had been consented to beforehand), thereby avoiding the cost of a second epidural.

While hospitals may be reluctant to undertake an epidural for ECV alone, it would certainly be worth requesting an ECV attempt before an elective caesarean, though you would need to discuss this in advance with your doctor. It is likely to be an unusual request and both you and your medical team need to be prepared for the two opposing possible outcomes: one recovering from surgery in hospital with your baby, and the other going home to wait for a head down labour to start naturally. You may also want to consider ECV during labour if you have an epidural in place (see below on ECV in labour and Chapter 10 on epidurals in labour).

ECV in labour

Dr Ranney (233) turned 7 of his successful ECV cases during labour and states that the prerequisites for this procedure are waters remaining unbroken, sufficient amniotic fluid, and adequate muscular relaxation between contractions.

Another small scale study looked specifically at the issue of ECV in labour (98). The hospital already had an ante-natal ECV policy but women in their study had not had previous ECV attempts; they were either found to have breech presentation in labour or had declined ECV ante-natally. They started the study trying ECV even when a woman's waters had broken, but the failure was so uniform with these patients that they continued only offering it to women whose waters were intact. They turned 11 of the 15 babies on which they attempted ECV, using tocolysis (with ritodrine hydrochloride). Three patients were under epidural anaesthesia. They conclude that ECV during labour should not replace the offer of ante-natal ECV but should be considered where no ECV has been tried (e.g., in the breech undiagnosed until labour starts). It is not clear why women with a previous failed attempt at ECV were not included in this study. This could presumably be another group who may benefit from another ECV attempt.

One study identified a group of women who were at particularly high risk of requiring emergency caesarean section – those admitted to the labour ward with a low cervical dilation, and suggested that these women might be particularly good candidates for ECV in labour (211).

Attempting ECV before term

As discussed above, it used to be the practice to conduct ECV earlier in pregnancy (around 30–32 weeks). This practice was abandoned for several good reasons, including concerns about the prematurity of the baby if the procedure precipitated a need for immediate caesarean, and the poor cost effectiveness of turning babies who might have turned anyway or might turn back to being breech again.

However, some authors have suggested that attempting ECV earlier is worthwhile, particularly for women with no previous pregnancies, who tend to have lower success rates for ECV because of the increased tone of their musculature (233, 203). Two of the people I interviewed said they would consider the possibility of earlier ECV (Donald Gibb (for women in their first pregnancy only) and Yehudi Gordon). Earlier in pregnancy the presenting part is not engaged and the uterus is less likely to be "irritable" (i.e., prone to experience Braxton Hicks style contractions during the procedure). One study did in fact find that ECV was successful in 74.3% of women who underwent the procedure at 30–34 weeks, while the success rate went down to 45% at 34–38 weeks (253). However, others have found that earlier ECV does not seem to significantly improve success rates (131).

There are significant pros and cons here and these need weighing up with your midwife and/or doctor. Realistically, given current guidelines from official bodies you may have trouble finding a doctor who is willing to undertake ECV before term.

Transabdominal amnioinfusion and ECV

There is one very small scale report of this method which essentially involves injecting the uterus with saline to artificially increase the volume of the amniotic fluid, thereby facilitating the process of ECV by creating more room for manoeuvre (22). The process of injection, which is done with continuous echographic monitoring takes ten minutes and ECV is conducted the following day. The amnioinfusion also has the effect of starting contractions but these cease within a few hours.

All six women in this study (who had previously had unsuccessful ECV attempts) had their babies successfully converted to a cephalic presentation. The authors suggest that the technique should be considered in women with narrow pelvises or with uterine scarring. I assume it may also be relevant to women for whom standard ECV is unlikely to succeed because of oligohydramnios (i.e. insufficient amniotic fluid).

This technique is clearly in its infancy and requires further evaluation. Because it is a relatively invasive procedure, it is unlikely to be offered at the present time.

EFFECTIVENESS OF ECV IN REDUCING
RATES OF CAESAREAN SECTION

The ability of ECV to reduce caesarean section rates may seem obvious. The ACOG states: "Clearly, women who have successful version have lower caesarean delivery rates than those who are not successful" (10). Factors which influence the size of the effect include the degree of spontaneous reversion to breech (likely to be higher in some racial groups (270)), the necessity for performing a caesarean section for other reasons, and the willingness of the local service to perform vaginal breech deliveries. If caesarean sections are routinely provided for breech deliveries ECV will clearly have a more significant impact on the caesarean rate.

There are studies which show no difference in the caesarean rate between women who have had successful ECV and women whose babies were head down in the first place (264). It is also not unusual to read in the literature somewhat cautious conclusions about the impact of ECV on the section rate, such as this one: "Even a high success rate for ECV only minimally reduces the overall caesarean section rate" (189). One reason for this is the apparently higher level of emergency caesarean sections in women who have had successful ECV which emerges in some studies. Why would women who have had successful ECV be less likely to have a vaginal delivery? One possible explanation is that babies who have been turned by ECV do not have much opportunity for their heads to engage prior to labour. It is also possible that babies who are not successfully turned may have been well engaged and therefore well prepared for a good progressive labour, enhancing the success of a vaginal breech delivery. Bearing this in mind it may be sensible, if you have had successful ECV, to practise any positional exercises which may encourage engagement such as squatting or crawling (see Chapter 7).

WHAT TO DO IF YOU HAVE HAD ECV AND WANT TO TRY IT AGAIN OR TRY IN COMBINATION WITH OTHER FACTORS

Because there are no policy statements related to good practice following one attempt at ECV, it is common, particularly in a hard pressed NHS, for this to be all you are offered. Many women feel that this is sufficient and it can form a starting point for serious planning for the birth.

> It didn't occur to me to ask for more ECV. Although I was really disappointed that it didn't work, I felt happy that we'd had a try and just wanted to get on with sorting out my care for the birth.

If you do want another try, the lack of clear research and policy in this area leaves you in a weaker position than you would be in if you had not been offered ECV at all, although presumably at least you may have a consultant who is in favour of it. The Midirs informed choice leaflet for patients says "If ECV doesn't work, you can have another go a few days later" (193). There is nothing to stop you discussing the options with your consultant. If you feel really strongly about it and do not receive support from your consultant, there is nothing to stop you from pursuing the route described in the last chapter for transferring hospitals.

SUMMARY

Factors which are reliably associated with successful ECV include having had one or more previous children (the more the better), and the baby's legs being flexed rather than extended. A scoring system is described which claims to predict accurately the likely outcome of ECV which you may wish to look at if you are trying to decide whether it is worth looking further afield for ECV. Interventions aimed at improving the success of ECV have varying success rates and may or may not be straightforward to access at your local hospital. Training women to identify any return to the breech position after ECV may be worthwhile for those small number of cases where this occurs. Tocolysis (using medication to relax the muscles of the uterus) may help, though not all studies support this so you may wish to have a try without it initially and may prefer to avoid the use of medication anyway. Having further attempts at ECV in itself should increase the chances of success. You may not be offered a second or third attempt routinely so you may need to ask for one. Fetal acoustic stimulation (where a noise is applied to the abdomen which makes the baby "jump") has been used with some success. Epidurals may help though hospitals may be reluctant to give you one just for ECV. You may want to ask for ECV if you have an epidural in place for an elective caesarean. ECV has also been tried in labour (though it seems not to be successful if your waters have already broken). Some people try ECV before 37 weeks of pregnancy, but this has various possible associated problems with it which may outweigh the benefits. Finally, a technique of injecting extra fluid into the uterus showed promising results in a pilot study, but is unlikely to be offered due to research being in such early stages. If you want to try any of these techniques discuss them with your doctor. If this is not successful, you may want to consider being referred on, though with some of these techniques it may be difficult to find someone willing or experienced enough to carry them out.

7
Self-help and Alternative Therapies for Turning Breech Babies

INTRODUCTION

This chapter tells you about all the techniques I have come across that aim to turn breech babies, other than external cephalic version. It covers acupuncture, hypnosis, positioning, homeopathy, chiropractics, Bach flower essences, and the use of swimming pools. I have started with those for which there is some evidence of effectiveness and moved on towards those for which there is no evaluation data available.

ACUPUNCTURE AND MOXIBUSTION

The good news for any of you alarmed by needles is that acupuncture's answer to turning breech babies generally does not require needles (although an acupuncturist may put in a couple to facilitate the process). Moxa is the Japanese name for an aromatic plant called *Artemisia vulgaris* (or wormwood) and is generally used in stick form. Moxibustion involves using the heat from burning moxa to stimulate the relevant acupuncture points. The point thought to be relevant to breech babies is the Zhiyin point (67) which is on the outer corner of the toenail of the little toe. Paul Clusker, an acupuncturist experienced in the practice of moxibustion, is quoted as saying of the approach:

> The site [the Zhiyin point] is not one traditionally associated with obstetrics or gynaecology but the action has been shown to be consistent. In my experience it appears to be effective and safe with no side effects when practised properly, which is why I feel it is worthwhile offering it as a way of reducing a woman's chances of needing a caesarean section. (9)

The standard application of this technique involves lighting a moxa stick and bringing it close to the skin until it produces reddening, though this should not be painful. The procedure normally lasts 10–20 minutes and may be repeated twice a day for several days. After an initial introductory session with an acupuncturist, you are likely to be given moxa to continue the treatment at home. You may well need to enlist support for this as you may find it is not easy to reach your feet! You may also be advised to lie in a position that disengages the baby during the treatment (such as that shown in Figure 7.5).

One of the difficulties acupuncture has, particularly in the West where its methods are not part of mainstream culture as they are in China, is credibility. "How on earth", you may well ask, "can stimulating my little toe influence the position of my baby?" The theory is explained by the Italian authors of a paper on the subject thus: "Moxa stimulation tones and warms up the yang of the kidneys, regularises their function and enhances the movements of the uterus and fetus, the position of which may thus be modified" (40).

The issue of scientific evidence for acupuncture, as with many alternative therapies, is a controversial one. Some have suggested that Chinese medicine may not be amenable to exploration by Western science (128) and argue for faith in its longevity: "The art of healing is thousands of years old. The science of healing is still in the process of being born" (88). However, particularly given the confusion about how acupuncture works, many feel that evidence is important.

There are two different types of scientific evidence on acupuncture for turning breech babies. The first relates to the proposed mechanism of effect; the second evaluates its success. Chinese reports suggest that there are statistically significant increases in fetal heart rate persisting even after stimulation of the Zhiyin point, along with some other measurable chemical changes. In a small animal study (15 rabbits), increase in contractile activity was noticed following stimulation of the Zhiyin point (40). It is not clear whether these studies used comparison groups to control for any of these reported changes that could have been due to chance or a side effect of being assessed (which can cause stress and therefore changes in the body). There is however anecdotal evidence suggesting that changes take place during moxibustion. The Italian group state:

The increase in fetal motility [i.e., the baby's movements]...is one of the more striking effects of moxibustion, perceived by almost all gravidae [i.e., pregnant women] toward the second half of the stimulation period persisting even after the end of stimulation. (40)

Much of the evidence for the success of acupuncture is anecdotal and small scale. This makes it difficult to assess the extent that acupuncture, rather than spontaneous turning, can take credit for any success. One example of this is a "success rate of 50%" for turning breech babies, quoted in an article on acupuncture in pregnancy (128). However, the acupuncturist concerned reports performing acupuncture between weeks 31 to 34 or 35. Since 57% of babies identified as breech at 32 weeks turn spontaneously (314) this is hardly an impressive result. One published study reported a success rate on a group of 100 women of 71% (68). Although this is higher than the rate of spontaneous turning from 32 weeks, the fact that this study included women from 28 weeks of pregnancy could account for this.

There is one highly promising Chinese study on the outcome from acupuncture with a good sample size and a control group (67). The results of this are presented in Table 7.1 and show that significantly more babies turned when treated by moxibustion than when not.

Table 7.1   Comparison of women who were treated with moxibustion for breech and women who were not

	Persistent breech	Baby turned	Total
Moxibustion	13%	87%	241
No treatment	51%	49%	264

Source: Cooperative Research Group of Moxibustion Version of Jangxi Province. *Studies of Version by Moxibustion on Zhiyin Points. Research on Acupuncture, Moxibustion and Acupuncture Anaesthesia.* Science Press, Beijing, p. 810, B19.

However, all of their sample were before 34 weeks of pregnancy, and it is not clear from the reporting of the study whether any of the babies turned back to being breech (as often occurs with early turning attempts) or whether the outcome describes the birth itself.

Edzard Ernst, professor of complementary medicine at Exeter University, remains sceptical about the success of this study and is quoted as suggesting that the practitioners may have given some other stimulus or advice that the control group did not receive (9). He states "I simply cannot think of a mechanism which could be involved. I would like to see the trial repeated in the west in the hands of more sceptical scientists."

The Italian group mentioned earlier attempted their own evaluation of moxibustion in 33 pregnant women (see Figure 7.1). Although their results do not look particularly impressive at a glance, and the sample size is too small to perform statistical analysis, their success rates are interesting.

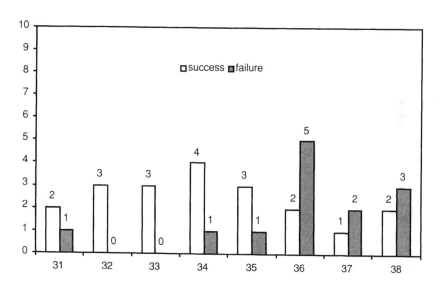

7.1   Results of moxibustion according to week of pregnancy between 31 and 38 weeks

Source: Cardini, F., et al. Moxibustion and breech presentation. *American Journal of Chinese Medicine* XIX(2) (1991): 101–14. Reprinted with permission from *American Journal of Chinese Medicine*.

The Italian group, despite their evident enthusiasm for acupuncture concluded, after reviewing all the evidence above: "It seems to us that no very clear answer has been given to the basic question: is the number of versions [turns] obtained with moxibustion greater than the number of spontaneous versions to be expected for the various gestational ages?" Some would regard this as an over-cautious conclusion and others would feel it is a reasonable interpretation of the available evidence.

One of the factors that may influence your own decision about whether to try acupuncture is whether you are suffering from any other conditions that acupuncture claims to offer help for, including nausea, high blood pressure, fatigue, anaemia, migraine, sciatica and backache.

People's experiences of moxa burning are mixed, though most are struck by its distinctive smell. "The smell was a bit off-putting – oaky and persistent, like smoky bacon" (9). Don't expect people around you to understand what you are doing and why. Some women's experiences of moxa burning suggest that you may earn a reputation as a wild, alternative eccentric (if you don't have one already). One woman had the following experience:

We burned the moxa in the garden so the smell didn't fill the house too much. Midway through a burning session, a neighbour stuck their head over the fence for a chat, took in the scene of heavily pregnant me sprawled on the grass with my partner waving a burning stick over my little toe, and rapidly thought better of it.

Another woman commented: "My husband thought I was a crank but he supported me" (9).

I have come across women who have faithfully burned moxa with no success, but also those who feel it has worked for them:

We will never know if it was the moxa that worked, it may have just been coincidence; but my gut feeling is that it did. My baby had plenty of opportunity to turn on her own so it's strange that it didn't happen until just after the [moxa] treatment. (9)

For help with finding an acupuncturist, see the contact details for the British Acupuncture Council in the Useful Contacts section at the end of this book.

HYPNOSIS

To my knowledge there is only one study relating to hypnosis and turning breech babies (190). This was published in 1994 and despite being a well designed study on a good sized sample of 100 women (and a 100 strong comparison group), with highly impressive results, I have not found reference to it since. Perhaps hypnosis has been so tainted by stage and television hypnotists that people simply don't take it seriously.

Dr Mehl, who is a medical doctor and clinical psychologist with an interest in birth, recruited 100 pregnant women whose babies were breech at 37–40 weeks. One third of his sample had already tried ECV unsuccessfully; 41% of his sample had had no previous children. He matched these women to a comparison group of women from a database who were of similar age, number of previous pregnancies, socio-economic status, race, geographical area and obstetrical risk status.

Women who had volunteered to be part of the study were offered up to ten hours of hypnosis (though a quarter of his sample had only one session and most had no more than five hours). They were also given a tape to practise at home. In the session, a state of deep relaxation was achieved and Dr Mehl then talked to them about breech babies. He described tension in the lower uterine segment preventing the baby's head from settling down into the pelvis, and suggested that relaxation would help the head to move down. "Trust in nature" and "Trust in your body" were phrases commonly used. The session finished with some self-esteem building suggestions.

An impressive 81% of babies in the group receiving hypnosis turned to be head down and remained so at birth. The comparison group had a conversion rate of 48%, representing a highly significant difference between the two. Dr Mehl does point out that the results in a randomly selected population would have lower conversion rates because of variability in motivation and suitability as a hypnotic subject. His own sample of self-selected volunteers were likely to have been well motivated which is clearly important to the success of hypnosis.

The difficulty in interpreting this study is to identify the key elements of the intervention. It is possible that the deep state of relaxation alone was responsible for the turning, by loosening the uterine and abdominal muscles sufficiently to make space for the baby to turn. The hypnotic suggestion element of the intervention may or may not have been relevant to the outcomes. Further research is needed to tease these elements apart.

Although Dr Mehl suggests that his research supports "a mind–body connection in the breech presentation", such speculations need to be treated with care. As discussed in Chapter 2, an intervention which converts a breech cannot necessarily claim it has addressed a cause of breech – the cause and the remedy may be entirely unrelated.

An extraordinary anecdotal account in Naomi Wolf's book *Misconceptions* is worth recounting here as it appears to indicate that suggestion (in this case not hypnotic suggestion) may be a potent turning tool (318). Naomi Wolf's own baby was lying in the breech position at seven months. The following incident occurred while she was lying on the sofa at her in-laws' house.

Before thinking, I blurted out to my relatives, "Hey, what if we all take a minute and send a request to the baby to flip around?" There was a beat of silence as my relatives considered my odd proposal. It was not the sort of thing any of us believed in. I have no idea why I came up with the notion – if anything suggested the idea to me at all, or whether my mind, or the baby's, somehow triggered some mysterious biochemical signal that future scientists will later be able to explain. Nonetheless, half a minute later, I felt what can only be described as a great lurching in my belly, like a lava flow buckling and shifting far beneath the earth. And our topsy-turvy baby, after developing mischievously head-up for seven months in no particular hurry to shift anywhere, since no-one had asked her to do anything about it, turned herself, properly upside down. (318)

Although this successful turning episode occurred relatively early when many babies turn from breech to head down, the timing of the baby's turning does seem remarkable.

POSITIONS AND EXERCISES TO ENCOURAGE TURNING

The rationale for most of the techniques described here is to try to free up the baby's movement and prevent the buttocks or feet from engaging in the pelvis (or tilt them back up if they have already engaged). They should be practised as often as possible, ideally at least on a daily basis. Since they all perform a similar function you may want to just select one that you find most comfortable, or switch between them to prevent boredom setting in. Many of the techniques can be worked into your routine – try them while you are watching tv, reading, on the telephone, etc., though you may wish to focus exclusively on what you are doing. Try to enjoy them and relax as you are doing them; relaxation is likely to promote turning and a little time out to relax may also improve your mood too.

Some people recommend additional techniques (though they could be used independently) to reinforce any benefits of positioning. These include talking to your baby as you are doing these exercises, encouraging him/her gently to turn. Visualisation (i.e., creating a vivid visual image of your baby turning in your womb while you are relaxed) is also a technique that many people regard as helpful. Some women have even shone a torch on their bellies in the hopes that the baby will follow the light! Evidence on all of these ideas is lacking. They are only worth doing if they make sense to you personally. If you feel daft doing any of them, don't bother!

The classic position is the Elkins knee–chest position, for which a high rate of success is claimed (see Figure 7.2). The woman kneels and leans forward until her head rests on her folded arms (so that the head is lower than the bottom). The knees need to be spread to make room for the abdomen. Elkins originally suggested that this was practised for 15 minutes every two hours of waking time for five days. In his study of 71 women with persistent breech presentation after 37 weeks of pregnancy, a remarkable 91% of babies turned and had a head down vaginal delivery (89a). In an attempt to evaluate the method in a randomised clinical trial, Chenia and Crowther evaluated the method in a sample of 76 women after the 37th week of pregnancy, 39 of whom performed a modified version of the knee–chest position procedure (only three times a day), with 37 women acting as a control group. They found that 41% of babies in the knee–chest group turned (and stayed head down) compared to 32.4% of babies in the control group (50). Though less striking than Elkins' original results, they suggest that the procedure deserves further evaluation in a larger study group. It seems possible that their lower success rates may have been due to the modification of the procedure – more frequent practising is perhaps better.

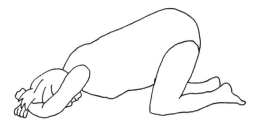

7.2   The Elkins knee–chest position

If you are planning to practise the knee–chest position, it is generally thought optimal to ensure that the first time you do it each day is before rising in the morning with a full bladder, as the slight weight of the full bladder is thought to encourage the foetus to turn.

It has been observed that there are frequent reports of spontaneous turning in several women immediately following an ultrasound examination to confirm the breech position of their babies. This has been attributed to the women rolling onto their hands and knees as they were getting off the examination table (92). Ilana Machover has integrated the knee–chest position and being on all fours into an exercise that involves crawling (179) (see Figures 7.3 and 7.4). Crawling is in fact recommended in the later stages of any pregnancy to help encourage the baby into an anterior position (i.e. with its backbone against the front of your tummy rather than your backbone) to avoid a difficult back labour (104). So there is therefore a double benefit to crawling. Although Machover uses the knee–chest position at the end of her crawling exercise there would seem to be some logic in also spending a few minutes in the knee–chest position before starting, to try to reduce the baby's engagement. She suggests that the best way to learn the procedure is with the help of a qualified Alexander Technique (AT) teacher. While this would undoubtedly ensure better attention to postural detail, this may or may not translate into practical benefit for turning your baby. The absence of a qualified AT teacher should in no way stop you from going ahead with the exercises shown in Figures 7.2, 7.3 and 7.4.

Specific positions for lying down with the pelvis tilted up also work in a similar way and are good, especially if everything else just feels like too much effort (see Figure 7.5). Juliet de Souza (49) developed the tilt position in Bombay in the mid 1970s. From the beginning of the eighth month of pregnancy, the mothers in her study were instructed to lie on their backs on the floor with an empty stomach, knees bent so that their feet were flat on the floor, with three good sized pillows under their bottoms, for ten minutes twice a day. She reported that 89% of 744 breech babies had turned to a headfirst position with this exercise, most within two to three weeks of starting it. As soon as the baby has turned, the exercise should be discontinued. This is a good sized sample with a remarkably high rate of turning. An informal account of the use of this technique was reported to me by midwife Alice Coyle:

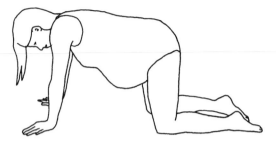

7.3 The all fours position

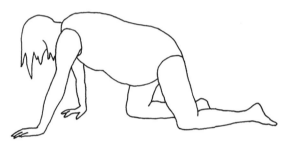

7.4 Crawling

A woman carrying her first baby which was in the breech position at 41 weeks went to Highgate Hill on a beautiful sunny day. She lay with her head down the hill and enjoyed the sunshine and the baby flipped around. She had tried ECV and acupuncture unsuccessfully. (69)

Janet Balaskas recommends asking your midwife or doctor which direction would be the easiest for the baby to turn and suggests gently massaging the skin on your stomach with vegetable oil in that direction (14). Gently is the key word here though; any force could be dangerous. This can be done while lying in the pelvic tilt position.

However, Machover points out two drawbacks to relying on lying down as a turning technique. Both the positions shown involve lying on your back: for women in late pregnancy this may be uncomfortable, and more importantly the pressure

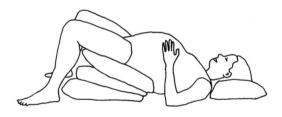

7.5 The pelvic tilt position

exerted on the vena cava (a vein bringing blood from the lower part of your body back to the heart) may lead to dizziness and fainting and can reduce the supply of oxygen to the baby (179).

POSITIONS TO RELIEVE DISCOMFORT

Breech babies can cause particular discomfort to their mothers due to the position of the head under the rib cage. There are various exercises designed to stretch the upper body/torso to relieve this discomfort. Annabel Hargrave, Active Birth teacher, recommends the following yoga positions: forward bend with partner, lying on back with partner, stretch and rock hips, lying on back with hips. Some of these are illustrated in *New Active Birth* by Janet Balaskas (14), and most yoga in pregnancy guides are likely to include them. Yoga or Active Birth teachers will also be able to show you how to do these and others (see Active Birth Centre contact details for a list of teachers nationally).

OTHER FORMS OF EXERCISE

Janet Balaskas also recommends walking for an hour a day to help turn a breech baby (14). This is based on the idea that the head is the heaviest part of the baby's body and will therefore have a tendency to move downwards, encouraged by the walking motion. Many women say that to walk for an hour a day at the end of their pregnancy is more than a little challenging, hindered either by fatigue or by bladder discomfort. This method of turning is more likely to be successful for footling breeches or breech babies who have not yet engaged. The engaged frank breech may well just become more engaged as a result of regular walking. In light of this concern, you may want to precede any long periods of walking you do with a few minutes in the knee–chest position or doing a pelvic tilt.

HOMEOPATHY

Homeopathy offers a remedy for turning breech babies in the form of pulsatilla. The standard recommended dosage is Pulsatilla 30x (a decimal potency), although 200c (a centesimal potency) is also mentioned. In homeopathy, the latter dose of 200c is diluted many more times and would therefore be considered more potent. Advice varies as to how long this should be continued, with one source suggesting that one dose every two hours for up to six doses is the maximum time period over which it should be taken. Others recommend no longer than two weeks. The concerns about taking a homeopathic remedy for too long relate to "proving", the process by which a remedy starts to cause the symptoms it is trying to alleviate. In the case of pulsatilla, which is also used in homeopathy to treat a whole range of problems, this may manifest itself as nausea or the production of a thick yellowy mucous.

Pulsatilla is thought to operate by causing the muscle fibres in the uterus to even out (321). However, there are no published studies evaluating its effectiveness. Sadly a planned study to do just this in a London Maternity Service foundered when it was blocked by consultant obstetricians who were not willing to cooperate (313).

Almost all books on pregnancy which suggest the use of homeopathy for turning breeches mention pulsatilla but recommend consulting a trained homeopath. However, it is not clear what advice a trained homeopath would have to add to this. There is no real choice of remedies to apply to the problem of breech (unlike most of the difficulties for which one might use homeopathy in which a careful assessment of the symptoms and personality traits of the sufferer is thought to be key to prescribing the appropriate remedy). So unless there is any other reason you may benefit from consulting a homeopath (and this may be worthwhile if you believe anxiety could be contributing to your baby's position (see below), or if you have any other troublesome pregnancy symptoms, you may simply want to go ahead and purchase some pulsatilla (from your local chemist, health food shop or other supplier).

The only other remedy I have come across being suggested for breech is based on the hypothesis that fear may be related to babies being in the breech position by causing tightness in the lower uterine segment. Ignatia 30c is recommended in such cases where fear is thought to be a problem (321) (although a trained homeopath might be able to suggest a remedy for fear that was better suited to you personally).

CHIROPRACTICS

The Webster Technique is now being promoted for turning breech babies (321). It was developed by the late Larry Webster, a chiropractor from Atlanta. A series of instructions can be found on the Gentle Birth Organisation's archives on the internet (see Useful Contacts at the end of this book). These are not for your own use, but to show to a chiropractor who may not be familiar with the technique. However, the International Chiropractic Pediatric Association recommend that a chiropractor should ideally see the technique being performed either at a seminar or on a teaching video, so if you are looking for a chiropractor you may want to ask them if they have done this. The technique is repeated every two to three days for two weeks or until the baby turns. I have not come across any published evidence of outcomes using this technique, nor any anecdotal accounts of its use, though this may be due to its being developed relatively recently.

BACH FLOWER ESSENCES

The only reference to the use of flower essences I have come across was at the Gentle Birth Organisation's website where someone had emailed the following:

> Someone told me about a doctor in Belgium who ran a maternity hospital who was also a Bach flower practitioner, who uses Bougainvillea flower essence for turning breeches, it was supposed to work really well. I just tried it and it worked amazingly fast. (321)

Anecdotal this certainly is, but if you want to try it you can obtain Bach flower remedies from health food shops.

THE ROLE OF SWIMMING POOLS IN CAUSING AND TURNING BREECHES

There is a rather confusing debate at the Gentle Birth Organisation's website about the role of swimming pools! On the one hand, there are many enthusiastic tales of the success of swimming pools, especially warm ones, in turning breech babies. The following is an example of this:

I always get my mom in a warm pool. [I am assuming this is an American Midwife talking about her "moms", rather than her own mother!] At least 72 degrees. She walks into the pool holding the baby's bottom out of the pelvis [presumably by supporting the lower part of the abdomen]. As the water gets deeper she can let go of the bottom of her belly as the water will hold the baby up. When she is up to her shoulders the belly is de-weighted and so is the baby. She should then dive head first down to the drain kicking her feet to help her get down. Water rushing by her stomach will help the baby to turn. I've never had this fail. One of my moms had to dive three times before the baby turned. The idea is that the mom and the baby are de-weighted and the heavy part of the baby (the head) will turn around. It also lets the baby decide which way to turn. Of course your mom needs to know how to swim. (321)

Handstands in water are also mentioned, preferably after 15 minutes of swimming so that the abdominal muscles have a chance to fully relax. The deep water immersion is also supposed to increase your amniotic fluid, which should also increase the likelihood of turning.

However under the heading "swimming pool supports breech presentation" at the website, the following anecdotal evidence is given: "I have dealt with four pretty stubborn breeches in the past two years and all of them were to women who spent a lot of time in the pool." There is then mention of three other women whose babies' turning to a head down position coincided with staying out of the swimming pool.

This apparently conflicting information is not necessarily mutually incompatible. Water is likely to have a predominantly disengaging effect, both by reducing the effect of gravity, and by creating relaxation which in turns provides more space for the baby to turn around in. If your baby is breech, especially an extended breech with a greater tendency to engage, a swimming pool will create an opportunity for your baby to move. However, if you use a pool regularly your baby may be discouraged from finding a stable lie, especially if its legs are flexed and it can kick itself round in all the extra space. So, my advice (based on speculation rather than evidence) would be to use the pool if you are not a regular pool user and your baby is well engaged and/or extended breech, and to consider using the pool less if you swim a lot and your baby has unstable lie or is a flexed breech.

SUMMARY

There is fairly good evidence that acupuncture (through heating a point on the little toe with a burning herb called moxa), hypnosis (probably through deep relaxation) and positioning techniques (particularly the knee–chest and pelvic tilt positions) may increase the likelihood of your baby turning to a head down position. Homeopathy (using pulsatilla), chiropractics (using the Webster Technique), and Bach flower essences (using bougainvillea) remain unproven but may also be worth trying. Swimming pools may be able to help turning and also prevent babies from finding a stable lie through their disengaging and muscle relaxing effects.

Part Three

The Evidence on Vaginal and Caesarean Breech Birth

8
Vaginal versus Caesarean Breech Birth: The Evidence

INTRODUCTION

The great debate of whether breech babies require a caesarean section to arrive safely in the world is a long running, emotive and highly controversial one. This chapter is not an exhaustive review of all the available evidence. However, I believe I have covered all the key papers of the last ten years, and also quote some papers from before this time. I have included quotes from people which are opinion and not necessarily evidence based, and hope it is clear when I am providing opinion rather than evidence. One of my concerns about the breech debate is that people often present opinion as fact, so I have endeavoured to avoid falling into the same trap myself.

The important message to take away from this chapter is that in many cases, there are few certainties about the best way to give birth to a breech baby. While this is stressful for you as an individual parent, weighing up the pros and cons of the options open to you, I also hope it will be empowering. In the absence of clear evidence pointing you clearly one way or the other the decision should become a joint one between you and your doctor and/or midwife. It should become more, not less possible to have your views and preferences for the birth taken into account.

I have decided to present the mass of data on breech birth according to the methodology of the study – essentially according to how it was carried out (with the exception of the section on premature babies which has mixed methodology). This means that the subheadings refer directly to the methodology. I have tried to explain clearly the terms used in each section.

My reason for presenting the data in this way is to give you the opportunity to think critically about what can or cannot be concluded from any given study and to understand better the limitations of research. However, it does not make easy reading and if you find it difficult to take in, the conclusions and summary should give you a good idea of what is covered. A consultant obstetrician reading this book prior to publication commented halfway through this chapter "This section is exhaustive and exhausting." If you find it too dense, you are in good company!

One key criticism which applies to all the research presented here and limits the conclusions we can draw from it is that all the studies describe medically managed vaginal breech delivery. Women are likely to have laboured on their backs, may have been given routine epidurals, had slow contractions speeded up with syntocinon, and had their babies delivered with forceps. The concerns about these various approaches are discussed in detail in Chapter 10. Although there are those who would regard this as a perfectly safe and legitimate way of conducting vaginal breech delivery, there are those who would regard some if not all of these interventions as actively dangerous. These people would argue that spontaneous active vaginal breech birth is the only safe way to give birth to a breech baby and that research cannot challenge the safety of vaginal breech birth until it starts to evaluate this approach rather than a medically managed one. To date, no such research has been done (although the historic paper on the Bracht manoeuvre discussed in Chapter 10 comes close to so doing with favourable results for spontaneous breech birth over medically managed breech birth (230)).

Another line of argument which casts considerable doubt over the conclusions of any study suggesting that caesarean section may be safer than vaginal delivery comes from a recent study on cerebral palsy, breech and mode of delivery between 1979 and 1986 in Denmark (161). Breech babies were slightly more likely to suffer from cerebral palsy than head down babies but the most significant link to emerge was between small for dates babies and cerebral palsy. There was no link between mode of delivery and cerebral palsy. What is significant about this finding is that smaller babies are more likely to be selected for a vaginal delivery, thus potentially leading to results which suggest that cerebral palsy is associated with vaginal delivery. This bias is a serious blow to many studies seeking to ascertain which mode of delivery is safest for breech babies (though it does not apply to randomised controlled trials where equal birthweights in each condition should be achievable (see below)).

Finally, a word of warning about reading this chapter. In comparing vaginal versus caesarean births, research results end up focussing on mothers' and babies' morbidity (complications) and mortality (death). These issues are difficult to avoid in the breech debate, but you may not wish to focus on them if you are late in your pregnancy and trying to think positively. You should find all you need to know for planning for the birth in the summary section at the end of this chapter and in subsequent chapters, so feel free to skip the nitty gritty of this chapter if you wish to.

RANDOMISED CONTROLLED TRIALS (RCTs)

RCTs are often described as the "gold standard" in outcome research. Following assessment, women suitable for either vaginal or caesarean birth, and willing to undergo either of these and participate in the research, are randomly assigned to either of the two conditions – a trial of labour or elective caesarean section. The huge advantage of this methodology is that it removes bias that otherwise could exist. For example, the vaginal birth condition will not include undiagnosed breech births who may have had inadequate ante-natal assessment and care. The caesarean birth condition will not include mothers or babies who have been assigned to this mode of birth due to ill health. It enables like to be compared with like, and the comparison should therefore be a fairer one. RCTs are also prospective which means the study takes a sample of participants and follows them up over time, rather than retrospective which involves looking back at care received. Prospective studies are generally less prone to bias and easier to interpret. They have the advantage of explicitly stating their selection and labour management protocols from the outset so that there is no confusion about who has been included and how they were managaed. The net result of all of this is that it enables us to draw conclusions from the data with some confidence, and make generalisations about what method of birth is favourable for which groups under which circumstances.

Surely all research should be like this?, I hear you say. Isn't the very point of research to enable us to draw conclusions about practice in a clear and meaningful way? In an ideal world, RCTs would be the norm. However, they are beset with practical problems. Randomising patients to different conditions is not as straight-forward as it sounds. Agreement from a number of obstetricians is required. Many may not be prepared to give it if they have already decided that caesarean is the best option. Many women, quite understandably, may not be willing to give up their own preferences about the way their child is born for the sake of research. Breech birth is relatively rare, and if one removes those women who are not deemed suitable for a trial of labour at the outset, the numbers are reduced still further.

Numbers are the main factor limiting an RCT. It has been estimated that to show a statistically significant difference in deaths from 5 per 1000 to 1 per 1000 a sample size of nearly 3000 women randomised to vaginal and caesarean birth conditions would be needed. If there is a small difference between vaginal and caesarean, it is possible that this would not show up in smaller samples. This needs to be borne in mind when reading about the first two RCTs reported below.

However, even in larger scale RCTs there is always the possibility that results emerge by chance alone. We may still be left with more questions than answers because it can be difficult to tease out which factors may have been responsible for negative outcomes. RCTs prescribe a standard protocol for large groups of women. If there are elements of this protocol which are controversial or with which we disagree (e.g., in the way a vaginal breech birth is managed), interpreting results can be limited by this.

Bearing these provisos in mind let us look in detail at the three RCTs on breech outcomes available, two of which are small scale, and the third of which is large scale and recent, probably representing the most influential study on breech birth to date.

Collea et al. (60) carried out a study of 208 frank (extended) breech babies after 36 weeks of pregnancy whose weights were estimated at between 2500g and 3800g, published in 1980. Of the 60 women who were assigned to a trial of labour, 49 delivered successfully. There were two mild brachial plexus (a nerve network in the neck and armpit) injuries in the vaginal delivery group that had recovered fully at follow-up. The authors commented that these appeared to have been related to poor delivery technique and were avoidable. They described as "striking and concerning" the degree to which women undergoing caesarean section suffered from infection, haemorrhage and unintentional injury (49.3% of the caesarean group compared to 6.7% of the vaginal group).

Another RCT was of 105 non-frank breech babies using the same selection criteria as above (119), published in 1983. Of the 50 women who underwent a trial of labour, 31 delivered vaginally. There was one neonatal death due to inadequate resuscitation, but the authors did not attribute this to the mode of delivery. This has been challenged by one reviewer, however, who suggests that the loss was preventable and should be attributed to vaginal delivery (259). He suggests that non-frank breeches are less suited to a trial of labour (see Chapter 9 on selection criteria for a more detailed discussion of this point). The authors of the study, however, concluded that the appropriately selected patient with a near term non-frank breech baby could undergo a trial of labour safely. They also point out that "The potential for injury to the fetus still exists at caesarean section delivery. Peripheral nerve injuries, bony fractures, lacerations and fetal haemorrhage have been reported."

The results of these two studies have been pooled and analysed together as one larger sample of 313 births (126). There remained no significant differences between vaginal and caesarean birth for babies' outcomes, and a significantly higher rate of maternal morbidity for women undergoing caesarean section.

However, these studies are not big enough, argue critics, to detect small differences in outcomes between the two groups. To try to address this, a multi-centre international breech trial was conducted by a research group based in Canada (127). Their results were published by Hannah et al. in 2000. They recruited 2088 women with a single frank or complete breech baby from 121 centres in 26 countries. Selection criteria used were fairly standard and included the exclusion of babies estimated to be over 4000g and women whose pelvises were estimated to be too small. The labour management protocol was fairly standard, and included permission to induce labour and to use augmentation and epidurals. They required that all babies were delivered spontaneously up to the navel with minimal inter-vention subsequently and no traction on the body. They did, however, permit the use of forceps to deliver the aftercoming head according to individual clinician's judgement. There was no significant difference in the weights of babies in the vaginal and the caesarean conditions. Their results showed that perinatal mortality (death at the time of birth), neonatal mortality (death up to 28 days) and serious neonatal morbidity (damage or complications from the birth and in the first 28 days) were all lower in the planned caesarean section group.

This study is regarded by many as sufficient proof that caesarean section is safer for babies, although those obstetricians I had contact with who felt the study left them with a preference for caesarean section continued to emphasise that, ultimately, mode of delivery was the woman's choice (123, 250, 293). However, as the debate about selection criteria and labour management protocols rages on, interpretation of the results are limited by disagreement over these factors. Critics argue that had the trial not used induction or augmentation of labour, epidurals, or forceps or had it used active birth positions, their results may have been different. In a table presenting information about the babies who died, induction or augmen-tation is present in 9 out of 14 of these labours – a significant majority. The authors did repeat their analysis excluding mothers who had not had an experienced clinician present (although concerns about the definition of this are explored below), prolonged vaginal labours, augmented or induced labours, and excluding breech babies with footling or uncertain presentations. They also performed a separate re-analysis excluding women who had not had epidurals, though it would have been equally if not more interesting to exclude those who had had epidurals, given the arguments advanced in Chapter 10. With these re-analyses, caesarean section remained superior although with a big reduction in the size of the difference between babies delivered by vaginal and caesarean routes.

One difficulty with interpreting the study comes from the level of experience of clinicians attending the delivery. The authors required an "experienced clinician" to be present at delivery which was achieved in a majority, though not all cases. "Experienced clinician" was defined as "someone who considered themselves to be skilled and experienced at vaginal breech delivery, with confirmation by the individual's head of department". However, when this definition was operationalised to include a number of years of experience, numbers reduced dramatically as shown in Table 8.1. Less than two thirds had more than 10 years' experience and under a quarter of clinicians had more than 20 years' experience. The low levels of very experienced birth attendants limits our interpretation of the results as we are unable to establish how different the outcomes may have been had more experienced practitioners been present.

Guy Thorpe-Beeston points out the difficulty with acquiring the necessary experience when breech is such a rare presentation:

At our hospital we currently have one or two breeches a month. Even if one person were to do them all [a virtual impossibility with shifts, annual leave and sick leave], it would take ten years before they did 100.

There is also the thorny issue of precisely what the experience is of, which will vary significantly according to the approach taken to vaginal breech management (discussed in Chapter 10 in more detail).

The authors analysed the combined outcomes of perinatal mortality, neonatal mortality and serious neonatal morbidity according to the level of experience of the birth attendant present. The results, shown in Table 8.1, show a trend of problems reducing as experience increases. When these figures for the subgroup of women attended by an experienced clinician are compared with caesarean outcomes the difference between the groups becomes dramatically less significant.

Table 8.1 Percentage of women attended by an experienced clinician according to four different levels of definition

Level of experience	% of women with a planned vaginal birth	% combined risk of perinatal mortality, neonatal mortality and serious neonatal morbidity
Experienced clinician present at delivery	97.3%	4.9%*
Licensed obstetrician present at delivery	78.4%	4.6%
Clinician present with >10 years vaginal breech delivery experience	60.0%	3.5%
Clinician present with >20 years vaginal breech delivery experience	24.1%	3.2%

* In the original article this figure is misprinted as an alarming but implausible 40.9%; 4.9% is my own calculation based on the raw data provided.

Source: Hannah, M.E., et al. Planned caesarian section versus planned vaginal birth for breech presentation at term: a randomised multicentre trial. *Lancet* 356 (2000): 1375–83. Reprinted with permission from Elsevier Science.

Another difficulty with interpreting the results is the standard of care provided by the hospital. The authors make the following distinctions between hospitals offering a "high" and "usual" standard of care:

1. the ability to undertake a caesarean section within 10 minutes if necessary versus 10–60 minutes
2. someone usually available in the delivery room to resuscitate a depressed baby, by giving oxygen by bag and mask immediately (versus within 10 minutes)
3. someone able to resuscitate by endotracheal intubation and positive-pressure ventilation immediately (versus within 30 minutes)
4. personnel and facilities on site to resuscitate and ventilate a baby requiring ventilation for more than 24 hours (versus needing to transfer the baby to another hospital).

Only 35% of hospitals in the study were able to offer a high standard of care. This is of serious concern as many would regard particularly the first two criteria of rapid access to a caesarean and immediate resuscitation (at the very least with an oxygen bag and mask) as non-negotiable fundamentals to the safe conduct of a vaginal breech delivery.

Analysis of the individual infant deaths in the trial also casts doubt on the study's conclusions (300a). Of the 2083 births in the trial, 16 babies died in total (plus another 5 who were excluded from the analysis due to lethal congenital abnormalities). Of these, 13 were in the planned vaginal delivery group and only 3 in the caesarean group – a statistic which, on the face of it, is convincing support for caesarean section for breech. However, on closer examination it is difficult to see how a significant proportion of the deaths in the vaginal delivery group could possibly have been related to the mode of delivery. One baby died in its mother's uterus, probably before entering the trial. It was also one of a twin. A pre-labour death cannot possibly be related to the mode of delivery. It is also somewhat bizarre that a trial which specifically excludes twins in its selection criteria includes the death of a twin in its analysis. A similar criticism applies to the inclusion of a head down baby, which also died in the uterus, probably also prior to entering the study. It seems even more extraordinary that this has been included as there is surely nothing to be learnt about breech delivery from what happens to a head down baby. Two more babies died after being discharged home well and dying subsequently. In neither case was a difficult vaginal delivery mentioned (though in one forceps had been applied to the aftercoming head). It is therefore difficult to establish whether the mode of delivery was responsible. Two more babies died from respiratory problems again with no mention of a difficult vaginal delivery, leaving us uncertain as to whether the mode of delivery was responsible or whether these difficulties would have developed anyway. Three more babies showed fetal heart rate abnormalities and in two of these it was stated that heart tones disappeared before a caesarean could be undertaken. Unfortunately the authors do not provide information on which deaths occurred in hospitals offering a high versus a usual standard of care, but the question of whether caesarean section could have been undertaken more quickly is raised. One baby who died following a difficult vaginal delivery was described as having "a small head, low set ears and deep set eyes" which is perhaps suggestive of congenital abnormalities that may have rendered it vulnerable. One baby who was assigned to the elective caesarean section condition died after a difficult vaginal delivery. The reasons for the failure to perform a caesarean as planned are not given, but one wonders when the plan of caesarean section was abandoned and how well staff coped with this change of plan. In terms of the management of a trial of labour this is hardly an ideal scenario. This leaves us with three babies who died after a difficult vaginal delivery. Interestingly, two of these had either induction, augmentation or both. As discussed in Chapter 10, there are many clinicians who would never use induction or augmentation and would proceed to caesarean section where labour did not start spontaneously or progress well. This leaves us with one death in the vaginal delivery condition that appears to be attributable to mode of delivery without question.

In the caesarean group, one of the three deaths was in a baby who ended up having a vaginal delivery (see above). If one examines the two remaining deaths in the caesarean group, it would appear that one of these was attributable to caesarean and one may not have been related. We are thus left with one death in each condition that is unquestionably related to the mode of delivery – a rather different picture to the headline figures. A more conservative analysis in the published literature recalculated the figure according to those deaths which could possibly be attributed to the delivery method and were left with eight deaths in the vaginal condition and two in the caesarean condition. This difference did not achieve statistical significance when analysed and therefore could have arisen due to chance (72a). Another perspective on mortality figures comes from an author who raises the issue of growth retardation (i.e., babies who are small for dates) (231a). This author points out that growth retarded babies do not appear to have been excluded from the trial and expresses concern about the ethics of this, given that allowing pregnancy to run its course (as would have happened for those in the vaginal delivery condition) would not be allowed in many cases of growth retardation, where policy is to consider section or induction prior to due dates. Growth retarded babies in the caesarean condition would therefore have been at a potential advantage in being born a week or two earlier than babies in the vaginal delivery condition. She suggests that seven of the deaths in the study were probably in babies who were growth retarded, and that this is a possibility for five others. The same author also points out that three deaths occurred in cases where intermittent fetal heart rate monitoring was used, and suggests that continuous monitoring may have picked up problems early enough to prevent a negative outcome (231a).

The measurement of serious neonatal morbidity has also been criticised. Paediatricians would have been responsible for assessing neonatal morbidity but they may not have always been available at caesarean section, especially in poorer settings. They were also not blind to the mode of delivery – meaning that the potential for bias (particularly bias caused by the belief that vaginal delivery is more dangerous) is present. The extent to which "serious morbidity" is justly named has also been questioned. How serious is hypotonia (deficient muscle tone), it could be asked, when it had disappeared within two hours in 7 of the 18 vaginally born babies? And what (if anything) is its long term significance if it persists longer than two hours? Another indicator of "serious morbidity" was "abnormal level of consciousness". In addition to being drowsy or lethargic, this category also included being hyperalert. What exactly is the problem with or the long term consequences of being hyperalert?

One very interesting finding to emerge from the study concerns differences between countries with low general perinatal mortality rates (broadly developed countries) and countries with high perinatal mortality rates (broadly developing countries). When perinatal mortality outcomes for the breech babies in developing countries were analysed alone, the benefit of caesarean section remained apparent. However, the difference between caesarean and vaginal delivery was no longer significant if results were analysed for mortality and serious morbidity combined in developing countries alone. This is in spite of more women succeeding in vaginal delivery in these countries (68.3% of women delivering vaginally in developing countries versus 54.7% in developed countries). On close scrutiny of the figures, developing countries appear to be performing rather better than their developed counterparts when it comes to vaginal breech delivery, and as Table 8.2 shows, this is particularly marked when the outcome of morbidity is studied alone. The rate of serious morbidity in babies in the planned vaginal delivery group in developing countries is just under half the rate in developed countries. Developing countries have less morbidity in more vaginally delivered babies.

Table 8.2   Babies' outcomes from planned vaginal breech delivery in developing and developed countries

	Perinatal/neonatal mortality and serious morbidity combined	Serious neonatal morbidity
Countries with high perinatal mortality (developing countries)	23/528 (4.4%)	13/518 (2.5%)
Countries with low perinatal mortality (developed countries)	29/511 (5.7%)	26/508 (5.1%)

Source: As Table 8.1. Reprinted with permission from Elsevier Science.

The authors suggest that if these findings are not due to some failure to detect morbidity in babies delivered vaginally they could be due to the greater experience of professionals in developing countries in delivering breech babies. This is one of a number of possible explanations for these findings. Another factor could be that the use of technologies such as epidurals, induction and augmentation may be lower in countries where resources and facilities are more limited. Sadly there is no analysis of the prevalence of these interventions in developing countries. It is also possible that psychological factors play a role. Because of the greater levels of expertise in breech birth it is possible that the "nocebo effect" (212) (discussed in Chapter 3), in which the anxiety in health professionals about breech birth is transmitted to the woman, operates far more in developed rather than developing countries. This possible absence or reduction in the nocebo effect may enable more women to have good progressive vaginal labours, helping more women to deliver their babies safely. The higher levels of successful vaginal birth following a trial of labour would support this. Although mortality figures would still suggest that caesarean section confers some benefit, there may be reasons for this other than the hazards of vaginal breech delivery, such as basic healthcare provision (5). It seems possible that if the same group of experienced personnel were responsible for delivering breech babies in a developed country, mortality and morbidity figures might show no benefit from caesarean section.

One obstetrician criticising the trial points out the low mortality rates found in a nationwide study from Sweden (174) and notes the trial's failure to match these mortality rates (278a). Surely the causes of this poor performance with breech should be investigated, he argues.

There are a range of other criticisms of the study in the literature. One critic points out that in some centres fewer than 1% of eligible women were recruited for the trial, although no systematic information is provided about recruitment rates and the total number of eligible women. In such cases of very low recruitment there is the possibility that bias is introduced through the small subgroup of women entering into the trial not being representative of the larger group of all women with breech babies (278a). Some have argued that the trial would have been more robust had more women's pelvises been assessed objectively (as only 9.8% of women underwent radiographic pelvimetry) (30a, 72a). Chapter 9 includes a detailed discussion of the role of pelvimetry in selection of cases for vaginal breech birth. Others have argued that the failure to assess the condition of the umbilical cord prior to labour was a serious omission from the study's protocol (297a). Technological advances in cord assessment mean that increasingly, some difficulties in labour can be predicted. These authors suggest that the use of colour doppler ultrasonography to assess the cord could have reduced the incidence of cord disorders and fetal heart rate abnormalities during planned vaginal breech births (297a). The same authors also draw attention to the limitations of estimating fetal body weight. A total of 91 babies weighing over 4000g were born in the study (59 of these in the vaginal delivery condition), despite the fact that the protocol stated that such babies should be excluded. This shows the inaccuracy of estimating a baby's weight in its mother's womb and the possibility remains that this high number of heavier babies may have affected the poor outcome in the vaginal delivery group.

In terms of women's outcomes from caesarean section in the trial, their results are unusual in that they showed that serious morbidity was not significantly greater for women undergoing caesarean compared to vaginal delivery. They suggest that "serious risks associated with caesarean section are fewer than previously described". However, critics would argue that comparing caesarean section with a medically managed breech delivery (where a woman may suffer morbidity from the use of forceps, e.g.) does not reflect the potential health benefit of a natural vaginal breech birth. The study does show longer hospital stays for women who have had caesarean section, but follow-up only lasted six weeks and so did not pick up any longer term differences in morbidity. Interestingly a subsequent meta-analysis of outcomes for women in all three RCTs showed a significantly greater risk of morbidity and mortality for women undergoing caesarean section (136). Risks of caesarean which have been demonstrated in larger scale studies than this one are described in Chapter 12.

Two babies born by caesarean experienced serious morbidity as a result of their delivery – one suffered a spinal cord injury and the other had a basal skull fracture. One critic points out that "even a caesarean section did not protect a breech fetus against serious fetal trauma" (231a).

Another finding to emerge from the Term Breech Trial is that in the elective caesarean section group, 6% of women still had a vaginal delivery because their labours started and progressed too rapidly for section to be arranged. This finding, along with the significant proportion of breech babies who remain undiagnosed until after the start of labour, make vaginal breech an unavoidable fact of life. The implications of this are discussed in the Epilogue.

One final perspective comes from the developing world, warning against the dangers of generalising conclusions from developed countries. James Erskine writes:

In the many less wealthy countries in which most of the world's population live and give birth, the availability of caesarean section is limited. Women may have to take long journeys on difficult roads, if and when transport is available. There can also be high financial cost. Surgery is not free to poor people, only to the well off or well insured. Facilities and expertise for caesarean sections on exhausted patients might not yield the optimistically low mortality and morbidity suggested by Hannah and colleagues [authors of the trial]....

The survivors of surgery have to deal with the prospect of the next five to ten pregnancies in their normal environment, hampered by the worry that their scar is going to rupture and require further, even more urgent, surgical intervention or lead to death. Some women who have had three or four children delivered, some of whom have died because of the high infant mortality in their countries, find that after the second or third caesarean, surgeons decide they must quietly tie the fallopian tubes to avoid future surgery made difficult through previous assorted scars. In The Gambia, the average woman is expected to have six or seven babies. To have fewer is commonly a source of serious anxiety or embarrassment, both to her and to her family. Loss of a child is a source of grief, not of shame. Loss of fertility is another matter.

Very few of the trial's collaborative group come from the resource poor areas of the world, where safe surgery is so hard to find.

Before the struggling nations of the world are shamed (unnecessarily) into inflicting a breech caesarean policy on their women, I suggest a major rejoinder to the article be published. Skills for vaginal delivering of breech babies must not be lost, and doctors the world over must continue to disagree with a policy of inflicting caesarean scars because it suits the practice of the richer nations. (93a)

The authors of the trial conclude that "the results of the Term Breech Trial provide us with reasonable evidence that a policy of planned vaginal birth is no longer to be encouraged for singleton fetuses in the breech presentation". While it is true that the Term Breech Trial provides us with the biggest and best designed research evidence yet, some may feel that their conclusion is premature. One critic argues that the conclusion of the trial must be qualified by the caveat "if managed under the protocol for vaginal breech delivery specified by this trial" (267a). He goes on to state that "This protocol would not have been acceptable at either of the United Kingdom's teaching hospitals at which I have trained", and specifies:

> Normal results on contemporary ultrasonography (excluding intrauterine growth retardation, excessive growth, abnormal liquor volume, abnormal presentation and fetal anomaly), spontaneous labour, rapid progress and a short second stage are considered essential prerequisites to vaginal breech delivery. A first stage of 18 hours, a second stage of three and a half hours, and liberal use of induction and augmentation [as occurred in some cases in the trial] would not be allowed. (267a)

The difficulty is that this may be the best research can give us. The likelihood of an RCT of sufficient size taking place that enables us to evaluate a more active approach to vaginal breech birth is low, certainly in the current climate. You may be willing to settle for the conclusion of this study in the absence of anything better. However, one critic has argued after highlighting the inadequacies in the data that "a policy of planned vaginal birth for selected breeches with a low threshold to proceed to caesarean section when problems arise may still be in the best interests of both mother and child". Many of you may feel that we are a long way off knowing for sure which is the best way to bring a breech baby into the world, and in the context of this uncertainty, make the decision which feels right for you.

LONG-TERM FOLLOW-UP STUDIES

Long-term follow-up studies aim to assess the differences in morbidity, or complications, in breech babies and the significance of these over time. They do not tell us anything about mortality rates as they only follow up babies who survive. Langer et al. (164) point out that studies assessing morbidity immediately after birth can include anything from an Apgar score[1] of 7 to major handicap and therefore fail to differentiate between major and minor problems. In longer term studies, significant handicap emerges more clearly and it is possible to test whether it exists more frequently in babies who were born vaginally. Unfortunately, many of these studies are about as retrospective as you can get in that they compare outcomes of interventions carried out many years earlier, although some studies prospectively follow up babies from birth until later in life. We generally have no idea of the selection criteria used to determine the route of delivery or the protocol for how the babies are born. However, it gives us some indication of the impact of the two delivery routes. Danielian et al. (76) carried out a long-term follow-up study, published in the *British Medical Journal* in 1996, of 1645 breech babies (at 2–10 years of age). There were no significant differences between elective caesarean

---

1. An index used to evaluate a newborn baby's condition, based on a rating of 0, 1 or 2 for colour, heart rate, response to stimulus of the sole of the foot, muscle tone, and respiration – with 10 being a perfect score.

section and planned vaginal delivery in terms of severe handicap or any other outcome measure. Rosen et al. (244) evaluated the outcome of 70 vaginally born extended breeches with a control group of breech babies born by caesarean section. They found no differences in outcomes between modes of delivery. Croughan-Minihane et al. (72) studied 1147 breech born children at 4 years of age. The route of delivery had no impact on rates of asphyxia, intracranial haemorrhage, neonatal seizures, cerebral palsy or developmental delay in the term or near term delivery.

Sorensen et al. (269) compared 164 Danish breech born adults with a control group of head down born participants on a measure of IQ. They found a small but significant difference between the groups, with the breech group scoring slightly lower (though many studies show no differences between the two groups). This difference persisted when the breech group was divided into vaginal and caesarean modes of birth, suggesting that caesarean birth conferred no benefit to babies' outcomes.

Sveningsen et al. (280) compared 709 breech babies born in two different time periods where caesarean section for breech had increased. Although they observed that the rates of a range of morbidity had decreased in between the time periods, suggesting that caesarean may have conferred some benefit, when they analysed the results they found that the improvement was not related to the route of delivery. This illustrates well a key area of confusion in the vaginal versus caesarean debate, expressed by Confino et al. (65): "Circumstantial evidence [has] emphasised the role of caesarean section in minimising fetal mortality." Because the increase in caesareans has occurred at the same time as improvements have taken place in other areas, perhaps most notably ante-natal screening and neonatal care, caesareans have taken responsibility for benefits that in reality would have occurred anyway, regardless of whether caesarean rates had risen.

Confino et al. (65) performed a follow-up of 93 breech babies at 2½ years and 8½ years of age, approximately a third of whom were delivered vaginally, and found that "breech presented children are similar whether they are delivered vaginally, or by caesarean section". Rosen et al. followed up 70 frank breech babies born vaginally, 70 frank breech babies born by caesarean section, 70 head down babies born vaginally, and 70 head down babies born by caesarean section for a minimum of two years (244). They found no impact of the route of delivery in relation to major brain damage.

A prospective study on an unselected group of 325 breech born babies followed up until 9 years after birth found that mode of delivery had no effect on neurological function (95). A retrospective study of 526 breeches found no difference in the vaginal and caesarean birth groups.

In their review of evidence on breech delivery and mental handicap, Westgren and Ingemarsson comment:

Vaginal delivery in strictly selected cases of breech presentation can be performed with minimal risk for the infant, and the rate of neurodevelopmental handicap will not be higher than in abdominally delivered breech infants or in cephalic presentations. (315)

Weiner (311), in his own review of long-term follow-up studies, comments: "[the studies] stand out in their unanimity. Vaginal delivery does not increase the risk of a compromised survivor".

META-ANALYSES

A meta-analysis pools a series of published studies and analyses the results as if it were one big sample. The obvious advantage of such an approach is that it provides far greater numbers than is normally possible within a single study. The main disadvantage is a variability, and often a lack of clarity about the selection criteria and management protocols used. The studies included can be retrospective or prospective. The outcome from a meta-analysis is only as good as the data that went into it, and if the validity of the original data is dubious, the results are too.

Apart from the meta-analysis of RCTs following the Canadian multi-centre study, the most recent meta-analysis is Langer et al.'s (164) study published in 1998. All the data collected came from obstetric departments with strict selection protocols and specialised medical care available at birth. Their sample size was 7239 breech births (just over half of which were delivered by caesarean). They found that there was no increased risk of mortality with vaginal breech birth. They did find an increase in risk for morbidity but argue that the wide variety of definitions of morbidity make this difficult to interpret, and draw attention to long-term follow-up studies suggesting that there appears to be no significant difference in long-term handicap between vaginally and abdominally born breech babies. Langer et al. conclude that "the process of resorting to caesarean section for every breech presentation at term does not seem defensible".

Weiner (311) concluded from his meta-analysis that "when good clinical sense was applied, the selected near term breech and term breech fetus was delivered as safely through the vagina as through the abdomen". He also pointed out that "cesarean section did not eliminate the risk of a traumatic delivery".

Stein (273) reviewed four studies comprising 2610 breech babies. He found no significant differences in mortality or morbidity between vaginal and caesarean births.

However, there are meta-analyses which suggest benefits of elective caesarean section. Spelliscy-Gifford et al. (271) pooled studies to form a group of 3056 women, 1231 of whom had a trial of labour. They found small improvements in babies' outcome for the caesarean group over the vaginal group in both morbidity and mortality, though they point out that "the risk of fetal injury in either case is small". Risk for mortality was not significant when analysed alone. They concluded "the potential increased risk of neonatal morbidity after a trial of labour should be considered along with the increased maternal risk from caesarean delivery". Their study has been criticised for choosing its criteria for injury arbitrarily (164).

Cheng and Hannah reviewed studies which included 12,278 women. Their conclusion, though apparently supportive of caesarean section is a cautious one:

The results suggest that planned vaginal delivery may be associated with higher perinatal mortality and morbidity rates than planned caesarean delivery. Because of selection bias in the majority of studies, differences in outcomes may be due to factors other than the planned method of delivery. An appropriately sized randomised controlled trial is needed to answer this question definitively. (49)

This study was criticised for including studies as old as 1972. Difficulties with data this old include non-availability of fetal heart rate monitoring in labour and ultrasound to detect major fetal malformations ante-natally, and the dramatic improvement in neonatal care which has occurred since then. It also has wide variations in inclusion of studies (both single centre and population based), making it impossible to establish what selection criteria and labour management protocols were used.

Bingham and Lilford reviewed studies published between 1974 and 1987 and found that vaginal delivery was associated with an increased risk of 4 deaths and 4 babies handicapped per 1000 compared to caesarean section (30). This risk appeared to decrease in the more recent studies to an excess risk of 2 per 1000 for vaginal over caesarean delivery. They spend much of their complex paper analysing the risk to mothers of increasing elective caesarean and set this against the higher morbidity associated with emergency caesarean section. On this basis they argue that the apparent disadvantage of maternal morbidity in elective caesarean section may not be as significant as the maternal morbidity produced by failed trials of labour that end in emergency caesarean. This argument is discussed in more detail in Chapter 11.

The difficulty with the variability in selection criteria in meta-analyses is not easy to address. As the authors of one meta-analysis put it: "Because each reviewed set of [selection] criteria is different and adverse outcomes in each study were low, we cannot identify any one criterion that may be responsible for an increase in infant morbidity" (128). The possibility remains that there are some methods of delivering breech babies vaginally which are more likely to lead to morbidity and mortality. These issues are discussed in more detail in Chapter 10.

POPULATION STUDIES

The major advantage of population studies is that they are very large scale and provide a general view of outcomes across a range of hospitals. They give us a sense of what is actually happening out there, rather than what is happening within a research trial. Population studies are always retrospective. So the lack of clarity over selection and labour management protocols which complicates the interpretation of meta-analyses is an even greater problem here. We simply don't know what, if any, selection criteria and protocols for management of labour were used. Invariably there is no access to the detail of the medical records of the participants concerned so it is impossible to know what circumstances poor outcomes occurred in and whether these were attributable to delivery routes or not. The presence or absence of experienced personnel attending the birth is not possible to determine. One important example of bias which could significantly influence results is the occurrence of intrapartum death (death during labour). A baby that presents in a condition suggesting that survival is unlikely, or who has died early on in labour, is more likely to be delivered vaginally so as not to risk the maternal morbidity following caesarean for an already compromised baby. There is an attitude in obstetrics which may not be immediately apparent to outsiders that a baby needs to be "worth" the maternal physical trauma of a caesarean. Stillbirth almost never occurs by caesarean section unless a mother specifically requests it. In addressing the issue of intrapartum death in population studies, Saunders attempts to dismiss the issue by saying that in one study, the fetal heartbeat was present in over 80% of cases when the decision was made to proceed with vaginal delivery (248). Given the extremely rare occurrence of fetal death, 80% is hardly high enough to reassure us that this factor is not contributing to the results.

Thus the danger is that large scale population studies are not in fact giving us the results that we really want to know about: they present unselected (or at best variously selected) breech birth, managed according to no specified criteria. We have no way of judging the level of experience of any personnel present at vaginal deliveries. The only bias which may favour vaginal delivery in a population study is the fact that high risk births are likely to be scheduled for elective caesarean, which could be expected to increase poor outcomes for caesarean (155). It is impossible to estimate the relative sizes of these various sources of bias.

Within the UK the biggest population study was carried out by Thorpe-Beeston et al. in 1992 (294). They studied 3447 term breech babies born within the North West Thames Health Authority between 1988 and 1990. They reported significantly higher levels of morbidity and mortality in babies born vaginally, with a 1% risk of neonatal mortality associated with vaginal delivery compared to a 0.03% risk for babies born by caesarean. This converts into a relative risk of 20 to 1 for vaginal delivery.

This alarming result led to a mass of critical correspondence in the *British Medical Journal*, much of it pointing out that because of the methodological limitations outlined above, conclusions could not be drawn about whether the worse outcomes for vaginally delivered babies could be attributed to mode of delivery or to other unidentified variables. For example, Paterson-Brown and Fisk of Queen Charlotte's Hospital in London suggested that the deaths may have been "attributable to problems unrelated to presentation [or mode of delivery] such as infection, abruption or intrauterine growth retardation. Certainly smaller babies are more likely to be selected for vaginal delivery" (222). Deans et al., writing from the West London Hospital, pointed out that

the group who went into labour are likely to have included those with precipitate delivery, previously undiagnosed breech presentation, and unbooked mothers who will be more at risk of a poor outcome. Any woman presenting in established labour whose fetus was found to be dead on initial examination would presumably have been classed as having an intrapartum death and been allowed to deliver vaginally....It would have been useful to determine whether a single factor such as the use of oxytocin or lack of senior staff in attendance could be implicated. To answer these questions requires a more complete description of the circumstances surrounding the deaths. (77)

Despite this and many other calls for a more detailed analysis of the eight deaths recorded in the vaginal delivery group in their study (27, 41, 155), Thorpe-Beeston and his colleagues have not subsequently provided an analysis of the circumstances surrounding each one, making it impossible to establish the degree to which they were related to the mode of delivery. Analysing the causes of death had a significant impact on the interpretation of the results of the multi-centre randomised controlled trial described earlier in this chapter. There is little reason to think that this would not also be the case for this study.

If the assumption is made that the excess in deaths in the vaginal delivery group was due directly to the mode of delivery, this would have been caused by trauma and asphyxia (suffocation), argued Paterson-Brown and Fisk (222). However, when one studies the rates of serious morbidity in the same study (as evidenced by admission to a special care baby unit), which should also show an effect of increased asphyxia and trauma, in fact babies in the vaginally delivered group were actually admitted less frequently (5.6%) than babies delivered by caesarean (5.9%).

Deans et al. also pointed out that the analysis should at least be on the basis of intention to treat. That is, the outcomes should be taken from all the babies who had a trial of labour, including those who went on to have an emergency caesarean section (77). When the vaginally delivered babies are combined with the babies who were delivered by emergency caesarean section, the difference in mortality between this group and the elective caesarean group is no longer significant.

This critique of Thorpe-Beeston et al.'s study shows us how cautious we need to be in interpreting results from research, especially population studies. Similar criticisms could be levelled at all the studies described in the rest of this section.

The largest of all the population studies comes from America (153). Kiely reported on 17,587 breech births in 1991, 6178 of which were born vaginally. This found significantly higher mortality rates in the group that were delivered vaginally. Krebs et al. studied 15,718 breech deliveries in Denmark between 1982 and 1990 (160). They also found that vaginal delivery was associated with higher levels of morbidity and mortality. However, they point out that a range of factors, other than mode of delivery could be responsible for the difference, including selection criteria, the structure of perinatal care or a need for improvement in professional skills. Roman et al. (243) analysed all term breech infants (15,818) born in Sweden between 1987 and 1993. They found higher risks of neonatal morbidity and mortality in the babies delivered vaginally. Two other large population studies (one of 11,000 (107), one of 9000 (246)) found a higher level of mortality for vaginal delivery, both in the order of 5 per 1000.

However, population studies do not uniformly support caesarean section. There are other studies which do not find a difference between the two modes of delivery. Lindqvist et al. (174) analysed all 6542 breech births in Sweden in 1991 and 1992. There were no significant differences in mortality outcomes and overall the mortality rate was significantly lower than in either the Danish or the British studies. Of the six deaths, two occurred outside hospital, two occurred in the vaginal delivery group and two in the caesarean section group. None of these latter four were felt by the authors to have been caused by the mode of delivery. They question whether their better mortality rates could be related to better selection criteria, or to higher rates of vaginal delivery in Sweden leading to greater expertise. The confusing aspect to interpreting this study is the subsequent publication of Roman et al.'s study above, suggesting that over a longer time period in Sweden, results may not be as good (243). In Slovenia, Pajntar et al. (219) analysed all 5012 breech births between 1987 and 1992. They concluded that the effects of abdominal delivery on the breech baby "are in many aspects poorer than in vaginal delivery". For a discussion of how caesarean section may adversely affect birth outcomes, see Chapter 11. Another more recent Slovenian study of 2952 breech babies did not find vaginal delivery to be a risk factor for poor outcome (231a). They had a caesarean rate of 30.4% and their mortality rate was less than ten (after excluding those babies with fatal malformations and those who died before labour). This mortality is no higher than what would be expected in head down births.

Acien (4) reviewed breech presentation across different centres in Spain and found no correlation between mortality rates and caesarean rates amongst the different centres. In another study by the same author, outcomes in breech presentation in Spain and Portugal were compared with those in Latin America (5). Interestingly, he found that higher rates of caesarean section did correlate with lower infant death for breech in Latin America. Acien concludes from his studies:

As long as basic healthcare is still an issue in certain countries, it seems that a high rate of caesarean sections could prevent or reduce perinatal mortality. Yet in countries with better health care standards there is probably no need to perform caesarean section in most breech presentations. (5)

The relationship between better outcome and caesarean in developing countries has also been found in other studies in South East Asia (170), Turkey (93) and Jordan (2). However, it is important to note that this correlation could have been due to an unidentified third variable. For example, women from higher socio-economic classes are more likely to have better health outcomes, and are more likely to be able to afford a caesarean. This explanation would explain the apparent contradiction between this research and the outcomes from the Canadian multi-centre trial suggesting that vaginal breech birth in a developing country is a safer option than in a developed country. The fact that the multi-centre trial randomised women to vaginal or caesarean birth conditions gives us a truer picture of breech birth outcomes in developing countries.

SINGLE CENTRE STUDIES

As with population studies, single centre studies are weakened by the lack of randomising, meaning that any difference between groups could be explained by differences in the make-up of the two groups, rather than the method of birth. They can be retrospective or prospective. However, the advantage of a single centre study is that it is often able to be very specific about selection and labour management protocols. Thus unlike in meta-analyses, population studies and long-term follow-up studies, we usually have a good idea of exactly who was selected for vaginal birth and what happened to them during labour. More attention is paid to the detail of selection and labour management protocols in Chapters 8 and 9 respectively.

The largest report from a single centre comes from the John Radcliffe Hospital in Oxford (180), though this is only available as a brief write-up as an audit (an evaluation of past practice) in the correspondence pages of the *British Medical Journal*. There is no information given on the selection and labour management protocols used, perhaps because the study was retrospective. The morbidity and mortality rates were not significantly different between the two modes of delivery for their 1946 breech babies. They report their perinatal mortality rate of 0.36% as similar to another study's (294) despite a lower use of caesarean (58% versus 72%). They point out that this mortality rate remains higher than that of cephalic babies (0.08%) and conclude that this is the case "irrespective of the mode of delivery and that some unrecognised lethal factor may be associated with [a small minority of cases of] breech presentation".

Schiff et al.'s (256) sample of 846 born in the period 1986–96 is based on a sample who have had access to modern ante-natal and perinatal care. Their study was "unable to demonstrate that perinatal mortality is significantly affected by the mode of delivery when selection criteria are applied". They conclude: "Consequent to the lack of reliable experimental data supporting a preferred mode of delivery for the term breech infant, the physician's decision is therefore more philosophical than scientific."

Daniel et al.'s (75) study of 496 breech babies is a good example of a well-conducted, single centre study. In addition to very clear protocols, the authors state that their centre had "a long-term tradition of delivering breech-presenting fetuses vaginally, including the nulliparous patients". There was no mortality in the study, and the authors found no differences in morbidity between the two groups. Of the 283 women who were deemed suitable for a trial of labour, 80% succeeded.

Albrechtson et al. (7) reported data on 1212 breech babies, 57% of whom were born vaginally. Interestingly, they reported their rate of emergency caesarean section for a failed trial of labour as 6%. They suggest that this low rate of caesarean section may be related to their strong tradition of skilled vaginal delivery, due to the presence in the past of the late Jorgen Lovset (1896–1981) as head of their department, who developed a manoeuvre to assist vaginal breech delivery (described in Chapter 10). They concluded from their results that "[No babies] died or had long-term sequelae [consequences] because of a complicated or failed vaginal breech delivery."

Brown et al. (36) report on the outcomes of 843 breech babies, although their protocols for selection and delivery were not specified. They found no difference in outcome between those babies delivered by caesarean section and those delivered vaginally, and suggest that their significant infant mortality levels (six babies died in their sample) were related to factors other than the route of delivery, such as prematurity and ante-natal complications.

Ismail et al. (143) studied 756 babies, 485 of whom were delivered by caesarean section. They found that poor outcomes were primarily caused by very low birthweight, congenital malformations and premature labour. The difference in mortality rates between caesarean section and vaginal delivery was not significant after adjustment for these confounding factors.

Irion et al. (142) studied 705 breech births, 269 of which were delivered vaginally. There were five deaths, all related to major congenital malformations and none related to the route of delivery. There was no difference in outcome between the planned vaginal delivery and the elective caesarean section groups. These authors also point out the significantly lower levels of maternal complications in the vaginal birth group.

Nahid (204) found that in 352 breech births, 32% of primiparas (women having their first babies) and 55% of multiparas (women having second or subsequent babies) could deliver vaginally with no significant difference in outcome between the two modes of delivery. A Mexican study of 104 breech babies, 75% of whom were delivered by caesarean, found no difference in outcome between delivery routes (though the numbers in the vaginal delivery group are small). These authors also noted 20.3% morbidity in the caesarean mothers, as compared to 0% morbidity in the vaginally delivered mothers (208).

Jaffa et al. (144) reported a prospective study of 321 women, all in their first pregnancies with term breech babies. Of these, 81% delivered vaginally with no perinatal deaths or significant perinatal morbidity. These "primigravidae" or "nulliparous" women are the focus of some controversy (see Chapter 9 for a fuller discussion of this), with some believing that they are more at risk of complications in a vaginal birth and others finding the opposite.

Barlov and Larsson (18) used a scoring system (reported in more detail in the next chapter) to select their sample for vaginal or caesarean breech birth. They studied 226 breech births, 45.1% of which were vaginal, and concluded: "It was possible by means of the scoring system to identify a group of women who could give birth vaginally, without any mortality or persistent morbidity." However, there is no proof that their good outcomes were due to the scoring system.

One two centre study from Holland and Belgium of 220 breech babies reports no impact of route of delivery on neonatal outcomes (79). The single case of neonatal mortality in a term baby was attributed to incompetence (probably on the part of junior medical staff) rather than the delivery route. There was also one maternal death in the caesarean section group which was anaesthesia related. In addition to noting the "conspicuously low maternal morbidity" in the vaginally delivered group, the authors also noted that infections occurred more frequently in the babies who had been delivered by caesarean section. This trial included non-frank breeches who were reported to have equally good outcomes (though the numbers are too small for proper analysis of this).

There are two single centre studies which find caesarean section to be safer for babies. One Turkish study of 1040 breech babies, 56.3% of whom were delivered vaginally, found significantly higher mortality for breech babies born vaginally (93). Koo et al.'s study of 306 term breech babies in Holland found greater morbidity for babies delivered vaginally even after strict selection (157).

Green et al. (124) approached the debate on the benefits or otherwise of caesarean section for breech using a different methodological approach. They carried out a study over two different time periods at one centre to assess whether the dramatic increase in the caesarean section rate between the two (from 22% in the decade 1963–73 to 94% in 1978 and 1979) had resulted in improved outcomes. They found no significant reduction in unfavourable outcome, although suggested that there may be a slight trend towards improvement. They noted that rates of asphyxia (breathing difficulty) remained almost identical between the two time periods, emphasising that "the risk inherent to the maneuvers of extracting a breech by caesarean section is similar to that associated with the delivery of a breech via the vaginal route". They conclude that it is possible to achieve satisfactory outcomes with a 22% caesarean section rate and that increasing this will not necessarily result in a reduction in poor outcomes.

A study in Greece of breech births in the years 1965, 1975, 1985, 1995 and 1997 was carried out and found that a "more than fourfold increase in the breech caesarean section rate was apparently rewarded by a twofold decrease in perinatal mortality" (182).

Oian et al. (215) conducted a similar analysis on their sample of 580 breech births. They divided their sample chronologically into those born between 1972 and 1975 when the caesarean rate was 8.1%, and those born between 1976 and 1979 when the caesarean rate rose to 32.6%. They found no reduction in infant mortality during this time, and indeed commented on a relative increase in mortality in the second time period. Throughout the time period they found that babies delivered by caesarean section fared no better than those delivered vaginally. Another similar study (280) compared the caesarean section rate of 16.9% between 1971 and 1974 and the increased rate of 37.1% in the period 1974–77. Neonatal deaths were the same during both periods.

These last two studies examining mortality over two time periods are powerful in that if anything one would expect improvements in outcomes over time due to improvements in neonatal care. The fact that no significant improvement can be shown does appear to be a particularly damning indictment of the move towards universal caesarean for breech.

It is interesting that so many studies in this section appear to favour vaginal delivery. It is possible that one factor in influencing this is that centres proud of their record of successful breech birth may be keen to set up a single centre study (e.g., 7). If this is the case, it may point to the power of experienced personnel in helping successful outcomes for vaginally born breech babies.

PREMATURE BABIES

The route of delivery for premature or pre-term breech babies is also controversial, and less well researched. Pre-term technically refers to babies born before 37 weeks, though in practice some of the studies of term infants already described above include babies of 36 weeks and sometimes a little younger.

There are no prospective trials of delivery route in premature babies. The occasional reports of attempts at conducting prospective trials for the pre-term breech baby have been universally unsuccessful in recruiting patients. An attempt to mount a trial was abandoned in America after recruiting only 38 patients over a five year period (324). A similar attempt in Britain, which was nevertheless published, recruited only 13 women over two years (226). There are presumably practical difficulties with recruiting women to such research trials. Premature births often happen without any warning and in a context of considerable anxiety, none of which is terribly conducive to entry into a research trial. However, there have also been suggestions that some of these trials have foundered because of the strength of support for caesarean section for the pre-term breech, and obstetricians refusing to enter women into trials because of this and medico-legal concerns (311, 23). Indeed, it has been confidently asserted that: "While there is variance of opinion about the best mode of delivery for breech presentation at term, there is overwhelming support for abdominal delivery in the preterm period."

The following statement in a review of issues around breech helps to explain the context for the stronger bias towards caesarean in pre-term babies:

> Premature babies are more prone to any trauma, and especially on their central nervous system. Supportive connective tissues [tissues which support the structures of the body such as bone and cartilage] and the skeleton are not protective enough to withstand mechanical trauma. Hypoxia (reduced oxygen supply) in the premature infant increases the risk of intraventricular hemorrhage [bleeding in the brain] and inhibits surfactant production [necessary to help the lungs function], resulting in an increased incidence of respiratory distress syndrome. (65)

Mechanical trauma and hypoxia are thought to be more of a risk for breech babies born vaginally.

So, what of the evidence? The same methodological criticisms described earlier apply here and should be borne in mind when reading about the following results. In the premature breech prospective trial mentioned above which was abandoned through lack of numbers (324), the authors commented that the only serious injuries occurred in babies who were born vaginally soon after arrival in hospital where supervision of labour was not possible. There were no equivalent injuries in the group who had planned and supervised vaginal delivery. Although the numbers are small, the authors point out that this could introduce bias into retrospective studies.

Support for caesarean section for preterm breeches has been shown in some studies. One population study in Holland of 899 babies born before 32 weeks found a significant reduction in mortality for babies born by caesarean section. In an older review of outcomes of studies of breech babies weighing 1000–1500g, the results appear to show a fairly consistent benefit of caesarean delivery, though the numbers are so small in most of the studies that it is difficult to judge the significance of this (65). All but one of the studies in this review were published before 1980 so there is the potential confounding bias of less sophisticated neonatal intensive care. In a meta-analysis of studies, caesarean section was shown to have a non-significant trend towards benefits in mortality risk over vaginal delivery (290), although the selection criteria for the inclusion of studies in the analysis was not made explicit. In a single centre study in India of 162 pre-term breeches, of whom 69% were delivered vaginally, a higher rate of birth asphyxia in the vaginal group was observed and a lower "take home baby rate" (309).

Other analyses have broken their sample down into separate birthweight groups. One American population study found lower mortality rates for all breech babies born by caesarean section, but found that this difference between the delivery routes increased as the babies' birthweight decreased (246). For breech babies weighing 1000–2500g the mortality risk was almost two and a half times greater for a vaginal delivery than a caesarean. In another study, 83 low birthweight breech babies were followed up in an Israeli hospital (116). They broke their sample down into babies weighing between 700 and 1000g and those weighing between 1001 and 1600g. They found no differences in delivery route for the lighter group but a benefit of caesarean for the group weighing over 1000g. To add to the confusion this data creates, another study found a benefit for caesarean in the birthweight group of 750–1249g but not in the groups below or above this (122).

One difficulty with comparing these birthweight groups is that the numbers in each group are low. However, one vast study of 371,692 breech births divided them into birthweight categories and found a lower mortality rate for caesarean in all categories which was highest at threefold in the 1250–1499g group and lowest in the 500–749g group (169). What is not particularly helpful about this level of analysis is that the chances of getting an accurate estimation of birthweight if you are going into labour prematurely are probably fairly slim.

There is also a significant body of evidence suggesting that babies being born vaginally fare no worse that those born by caesarean section. In an American study of 262 babies born weighing less than 1500g the authors were able to tease out the effects of degree of prematurity and weight of the baby from mode of delivery (55). They concluded that other factors (such as low birthweight) were responsible for the poor outcomes of premature breech babies, rather than the breech presentation itself, and that the route of delivery did not significantly influence outcomes for extended and complete breeches. However, they did suggest that caesarean may offer benefit for footling breeches.

A recently published Dutch study compared breech babies born between 26 and 31 weeks from one centre which favoured caesarean delivery for this group, with babies from another centre favouring vaginal delivery. Their outcome measure was survival without disability or handicap and they found no difference between the two centres. In an Indian study of 224 breech babies born between 28 and 36 weeks of pregnancy, there was no difference in the outcomes between vaginally and caesarean delivered babies (183). Similarly, Emembolu (91) did not find a statistically significant difference in the mortality of low birthweight breech infants born vaginally or by caesarean. A study from North Jordan of 98 breech babies delivered between 26 and 36 weeks, 32 of whom were delivered by caesarean, concluded: "even with optimum neonatal care facilities, caesarean section does not offer any advantage over vaginal delivery in a developing country" (323).

Effer et al. reviewed evidence in Canadian low birthweight breeches between 1976 and 1980 (87). They pointed out that the increase in caesarean rate in this period from 11.9% to 49.1% was assumed to be responsible for the drop in mortality by 20% in low birthweight breeches in the same time frame. However, by looking at the mortality rates in head down babies in the same period, they were able to show that similar reductions in mortality had occurred without any significant rise in caesarean rate. They point out that

> the increased caesarean section rate may be incidental and in no way related to the improved outcome [in premature breeches]....We are greatly concerned about authors who in recent publications admit to deficiencies in the evidence that they present and yet conclude that caesarean section is the method of choice for delivery of the very low birth weight breech infant.

They conclude: "As yet unidentified perinatal care practices, other than caesarean section may be more likely to affect outcome in this high risk group."

Another study finding no benefit from caesarean section looked at the specific outcome of head entrapment, and the consequences of it, in 321 breech babies born between 28 and 36 weeks of pregnancy (241). Head entrapment refers to difficulty in delivery of the head of a breech baby. Head entrapment is an oft-cited reason for avoiding vaginal breech delivery. It has been argued that the chances of it occurring in a term breech baby are minimal as the diameter of the baby's body (and especially the combined diameter of legs and body in an extended or complete breech) is not significantly different (252). However this leaves open the possibility that head entrapment is a significant risk with the premature baby. The results of this American study explode three myths about head entrapment in the premature breech baby. The first of these is on rates of head entrapment, which occurred in 5.2–7.7% of babies. Although this is not an insignificant proportion, the prevalence of head entrapment in premature babies is not as high as some more alarmist commentators might suggest. The second myth exploded by the study is that head entrapment is the exclusive domain of the vaginal delivery. The study found that head entrapment was as likely to occur in caesarean birth as it was in vaginal birth. The third myth is of the supposed catastrophic outcome of head entrapment. The authors describe various approaches to managing head entrapment, including the use of medication to aid uterine relaxation, and conclude: "those neonates who did experience head entrapment with either method of delivery did not appear to have more adverse outcomes than those neonates who did not have entrapped heads".

Interestingly there is a survey of consultant obstetricians' views on the delivery of the preterm breech baby in England and Wales, published in 1991 (225). They found that 76% of respondents used caesarean section for the pre-term breech (though only 12% would for very premature babies of less than 26 weeks). This is in spite of the fact that only 35% of respondents thought that there was sufficient evidence to support such a practice. Only 12% would deliver a head down premature baby by caesarean section. Overall, 71% said they were affected by medico-legal considerations in their management of the pre-term breech. The conclusion by the study's authors is worth noting:

> These results demonstrate that a management policy does not have to be scientifically validated before it is taken up into clinical orthodoxy (and later, the obstetric textbook). There may be a belief that in a difficult situation any obstetric

intervention is better than none, even when it is of no proven benefit. This is likely to be particularly true when there are medico-legal pressures and masterly inactivity may be seen as neglect.

Thus regardless of the conflicting and confusing evidence presented above, the likelihood is, at least for a premature baby in England and Wales, that you will be offered caesarean section.

ANALYSIS OF REASONS FOR DEATHS OF BREECH BABIES

A recent article in the *British Medical Journal* reported on findings from the seventh annual Confidential Enquiry into Stillbirths and Deaths in Infancy (64). It states: "The single and most avoidable factor in causing stillbirths and deaths among breech babies is suboptimal care given in labour." Hypoxia (or oxygen deprivation) before delivery was the most common cause of death and delays in response to evidence of fetal distress occurred in nearly three quarters of cases. Delays ranged from 30 minutes to 10 hours. What is interesting about the findings is that they suggest that the risk to a baby from vaginal breech labour comes from the management of it rather than factors inherent in the process itself. The implication is that many (if not all) the deaths were preventable. Various recommendations are made in the report including training in vaginal breech delivery for all staff, training in the use and interpretation of fetal monitoring and that "trusts should ensure that the most experienced available practitioner is involved and present at a vaginal breech delivery". The management of vaginal breech birth is discussed in detail in Chapter 10.

CONCLUSIONS

The decision about route of delivery for the breech baby has been termed a conundrum (90). Just as the studies produce some results which support caesarean as the safer option and others which do not, so too do the conclusions from this research. This section presents a handful of conclusions to help you start to think about how to pull together what you have read in this chapter. The authors of one paper concluded:

Considering the contradictory evidence on the basis of which many mothers all over the world are subjected to caesarean section for an infant presenting by the breech, the ethical justification of such a policy is questionable. (23)

A similar point was made by the authors of a meta-analysis in 1998: "the practice of resorting to caesarean section for every breech presentation of 34 weeks or more does not seem defensible today" (164). Another author commented:

The sad fact is that babies in the breech position are at higher risk than cephalic babies. Unfortunately widespread use of caesarean delivery for breech babies has not demonstrated an improvement in the outcome statistics. Caesarean operations do not guarantee delivery of healthy babies, breech or otherwise.

Weiner, in his review of the evidence on breech delivery, concludes:

routine caesarean delivery of the near-term or term breech fetus increases maternal morbidity, maternal mortality and the cost to society, but it does not provide a forseeable benefit to the near-term and term breech fetus....Although preached with great emotion, the recommendation for routine elective caesarean section to deliver the near-term or term breech fetus cannot be substantiated by studies published over the last decade. (311)

The increased morbidity for women of caesarean section comes out consistently in almost all the studies.[2] Complications are often thought to be minor infections, and nothing to become overly concerned about. However, some authors point out that this morbidity "may be severe and includes hysterectomy, sepsis, and incisions which encroached on the upper segment of the uterus with consequences for subsequent pregnancies" (290).

These same authors offer a perspective on the decision making around birth showing that it should not be solely considerations about the baby that figure. They suggest that the choice, even for the premature baby, is "still finely balanced" and describe one of the author's opinions as follows: "R.J.L....believed...that caesarean section was probably a little safer for the baby, but would have advised that the modest and uncertain gain might not justify the maternal hazards" (290).

Since the Term Breech Trial, many people have assumed that we finally have the evidence we need to recommend caesarean delivery for breech babies. The authors of the trial summarise: "We have shown that a policy of planned caesarean section is substantially better for the singleton fetus in the breech presentation at term." One reviewer commenting on the methodological problems dogging all other studies on the issue said: "The international term breech trial was designed to reduce the uncertainty [about the best way to bring a breech baby into the world] and it certainly did" (177). However, depending on your view of the criticisms of the study, you may not agree.

One of the interesting issues in looking at the mortality and morbidity outcomes is the wide spread of results across the studies. It is not unusual to see clusters of mortality and morbidity in a single study (268), alongside other studies showing little or no mortality and morbidity (7, 60). The evidence from the Term Breech Trial on the lower rates of morbidity in developing countries suggests that higher levels of skill and experience may influence outcomes. The conclusion from the analysis of deaths of breech babies that "the single and most avoidable factor in causing stillbirths and deaths among breech babies is suboptimal care given in

---

2. The greater mortality risk to mothers from caesarean section is not brought out in this chapter because large scale studies are required. Chapter 12 reports research suggesting that the mortality risk is three to seven times greater for caesarean over vaginal birth.

labour" is also strongly suggestive that the quality and experience of the personnel managing a vaginal labour is critical.

SUMMARY

This chapter examines outcome studies comparing vaginal and caesarean breech birth and presents them according to the design of the study. This is to draw attention to the strengths and limitations of different research designs. Of the best designed studies (randomised controlled trials), two smaller ones, one on frank and the other on non-frank breeches, suggest no differences in outcome between vaginal and caesarean birth. However, the largest study to date – the Term Breech Trial – conducted across several centres throughout the world found that babies were significantly less likely to suffer morbidity or mortality from caesarean section than from vaginal delivery. Many obstetricians regard this study as significant justification for a policy of recommending routine caesarean section for breech. Critics argue that because it only evaluates a medical approach to breech birth it cannot dismiss the potential value of spontaneous breech birth (discussed more in Chapter 10). There are also questions about the extent to which many of the negative outcomes in the vaginally delivered breech group were attributable to the route of delivery or to other unrelated factors.

Long-term follow-up studies unanimously show no difference in outcome several years after birth. Results from meta-analyses (which pool several studies and analyse their results together), population studies and single centre studies are mixed, with some suggesting benefits to caesarean and others suggesting no difference. All these studies are particularly difficult to interpret because of various possible sources of bias. There is similar confusion over the management of premature babies in the breech position, with mixed evidence as to which mode of delivery is best. Survey data suggest that most obstetricians nevertheless tend to opt for caesareans.

Almost all studies show that caesareans produce worse outcomes for mothers. It is this factor which leads some people to argue that if vaginal breech birth can be shown to be as safe as, or even only slightly riskier than caesarean breech birth, it is the most sensible route of delivery.

Depending on your reading of the Term Breech Trial, we are left with considerable uncertainty about the best way to bring a breech baby into the world. One reason for the variable and contradictory results presented in this chapter may be differences in expertise and delivery technique at different institutions. Thus excess morbidity and mortality for vaginal breech birth could be caused by preventable factors. The implications of this for you and for services are explored in Part Four and the Epilogue.

It would perhaps be most sensible to conclude that vaginal breech birth could be as safe as caesarean section in the right place with the right birth attendants. Where you have your baby and who with may be more important than which delivery route you choose. Part Four of this book aims to help you research the options open to you and lists questions you can ask to try to establish the level of expertise and experience available. All women should have the right to access skilled and experienced birth attendants for a vaginal breech birth. However, this is a vision, not a reality. For as long as we have patchy and inconsistent services, the onus is on you to consider the evidence above and work out the options open to you.

9
Selection Criteria for Vaginal Breech Birth

INTRODUCTION

Selection criteria could equally be labelled exclusion criteria – their purpose is one and the same. Selection criteria are at the heart of many arguments for a trial of vaginal delivery. "Vaginal delivery is safe in selected cases of breech" is an oft-heard cry in obstetric circles supporting a vaginal delivery of breech. However, there are very few of the commonly used selection criteria which are well supported by evidence. Most would argue that they are securely based in good clinical judgement, though from the discussion below you may conclude that this is more so for some criteria than for others. One critic observed that "most selection criteria seem to have arisen through retrospective analysis of cases where a bad outcome was seen and assumptions were made as to the causation" (249). He goes on to point out that the application of a rigorous selection protocol will exclude a large proportion of women from even attempting to give birth.

Evidence casting doubt on the value of selection criteria comes from studies which show that "undiagnosed" breeches (i.e., those undiagnosed until labour has started) fare as well as those who have had the supposed benefit of ante-natal assessment and selection (59, 211), and in some studies are far more likely to have a successful vaginal delivery (42% of undiagnosed breeches having a vaginal delivery versus only 11% of diagnosed breeches in one study (171)). However, the babies in these studies were often subject to some form of last minute selection process carried out in the first stage of labour so this cannot be used to dismiss the worth of selection criteria entirely. There is also recent evidence from the seventh report from the Confidential Enquiry into Stillbirths and Deaths in Infancy (64) that suggests that undiagnosed breeches may be at particular risk. However, the fact that they include in their analysis all babies weighing over 1500g means that prematurity could be confounding their results (i.e., premature babies are more likely to arrive unexpectedly, more likely to be undiagnosed and more likely to have problems as a result of their prematurity).

Leaving clinical judgement to one side, the medico-legal climate is such that most obstetricians are likely to use a list of criteria prior to labour to select or exclude you from a trial of labour. If you feel unhappy about being excluded from a trial of labour, the chances are you will be on relatively strong territory to argue your case (see Chapter 13 on negotiating). There are many experts in the field who argue that a good progressive first stage of labour is the best, and in some cases the only selection criterion necessary. This is discussed at the end of this chapter.

POSITION OF THE BABY

Hyperextension of the baby's head

Hyperextension of the head in a breech baby is sometimes termed "stargazer breech". Rather than having its chin tucked into its chest, the baby has its head upright or stretched back. It is reported to occur in approximately 5% of breech presentations, though definitions vary according to the degree of hyperextension (some suggesting greater than 90 degrees, others suggesting 105 degrees) (259). However, three of the people I spoke to (Wendy Savage, Michel Odent and Donald Gibb) had not seen any cases of hyperextension of the neck, despite having seen many hundreds of breech babies. Wendy Savage reported that a colleague from Sweden had audited their figures and found an incidence of far lower than 5%.

The cause is often unknown but can sometimes be related to the cord being around the neck, congenital hypertonus (excessive tension) of the neck muscles, a cyst in the neck or fetal goitre (an enlarged thyroid gland causing a swelling in the front of the neck). Ultrasound is the most reliable way of identifying hyperextension of the baby's head.

This is the one selection critieria on which obstetricians and midwives would almost unanimously agree to be a clear indication for caesarean. The risk is of spinal cord injury during vaginal delivery and estimates of the likelihood of damage are chillingly high. Studies report 25%–70% of babies with hyperextended heads experiencing spinal cord damage when born vaginally, with 70% of those babies who were damaged dying as a result. The long-term outcome of those babies who are delivered safely is reported to be excellent, though the hyperextension can persist for several weeks post-natally, depending on the cause (259).

Extended (frank) breech

The extended breech has had the most favourable outcomes in most studies with many investigators suggesting that there is no difference in mortality rates to head down babies and serious morbidity of only 0–2% (53, 102, 60). In a survey of Canadian obstetricians in 1996, almost all the respondents supported a trial of labour for a term frank breech presentation (224).

Flexed (complete and footling) breech

The complete breech is seen as next most favourable after frank, with footling presentations being least favourable for vaginal delivery. For some the flexed breech is seen as sufficient indication for caesarean, others will permit a trial of labour to complete breeches but not footlings, and still others regard neither as grounds for exclusion. The two are considered together here as the literature tends to lump them together and also because some complete breeches change into a footling breech as labour progresses (79).

One concern about flexed breeches is that the presenting part – generally the feet, or feet and bottom combined – is not such a good fit for the cervix as the bottom is in the extended breech or the head is in a head down birth. This increases the risk of cord prolapse, where the umbilical cord falls through the cervix when the waters break and becomes squashed below the baby, risking cutting off its oxygen supply. Emergency caesarean section would normally follow. The prevalence of the problem of cord prolapse in flexed breeches is estimated to be at around 10%. However, some authors make a convincing case for not over-reacting to the possibility of cord prolapse.

Cord prolapse does not occur in 90% of these cases [i.e., flexed breeches]; when it does occur it is normally associated with good fetal outcome. Cord prolapse in the nonfrank [flexed] breech presentation, although an indication for caesarean delivery, usually does not have as severe an outcome as in vertex [head down] or frank breech presentations. Because the cord is prolapsed between the fetal legs, it is often not markedly compressed during subsequent contractions. (287)

Wendy Savage echoes this point, pointing out that cord prolapse is "not such a desperate emergency as it is in a head down presentation where the head comes down like a cork in a bottle....it isn't an immediate cut off of the blood supply and you've got time to take the mum to theatre and do a caesar if she's not fully dilated". This is supported by research which suggests that the same factors which predispose the baby to cord prolapse also protect it from becoming completely squashed (245).

Another concern about flexed breeches is the tendency for the feet to slip down through the cervix before dilation is complete. This can give the woman the urge to push prematurely and can lead to entrapment of the head if not managed properly. However, with an experienced midwife or obstetrician to assess the degree of dilation, the urge to push can be controlled, either using panting in the knee–chest position (see Chapter 7) or an epidural (see Chapter 10 for a more detailed discussion of epidurals).

The only trial specifically of non-frank breech babies was prospective and randomised, though small (105 babies, of whom only 35 were born vaginally) (119). This study failed to find any benefit of caesarean section in terms of morbidity or mortality, though it did have a 10% rate of either cord or body prolapse through an incompletely dilated cervix. Other studies which have included non-frank breeches have presented a mixed picture, some finding no worse outcomes for complete breeches (18, 79) but one reporting worse outcomes (245).

The Canadian Consensus on Breech Management at Term (284) and the FIGO Committee on Perinatal Health (163) both recommend caesarean section for footling breeches.

NUMBER OF PREVIOUS PREGNANCIES (PARITY)

Parity is divided into two categories: nulliparity, or no previous pregnancies (sometimes referred to as primiparity or a primigravida to describe the woman carrying her first baby), and multiparity, or one or more previous pregnancies (or multigravida to describe the woman).

The relevance of parity to selecting candidates for vaginal breech birth is a hotly debated topic with some arguing that nulliparity should exclude a woman from a trial of labour, and a few arguing that in fact multiparity makes vaginal breech labour less safe.

The argument against nulliparous women having a trial of labour rests on the idea that a woman with no previous birth history has an "unproven" or untested pelvis. In the pessimistic world of obstetrics, this "not knowing" is tantamount to being high risk – hence the exclusion of some women from a trial of labour on the grounds of nulliparity.

Karp criticises this approach to parity, and his description of the decision making process is worth documenting in full:

> Most obstetricians will permit at least some of their multiparous patients with breech presentations to undertake a trial of labour, yet at the mere mention of the words "primigravida breech" these same physicians grab frantically for the nearest scalpel. Why this peculiar dichotemous behaviour? "Well" goes the usual explanation, "its because the 'multip' has a proved pelvis"....But of what, precisely, has the multip's pelvis been proved? (149)

He goes on to point out that in a normal head down birth the head is so moulded by the process that its dimensions will be smaller than the dimensions of the head of a breech baby. He also says that head size increases with parity. Thus the evidence of a previous birth with no problems does not offer the level of reassurance that those who exclude nulliparous women from a trial of labour would suggest that it does. Karp concludes that "all breech presentations must be accorded equal respect" and that "The concept of a proved pelvis in relation to a breech presentation should be recognised as the myth it has become."

The evidence on parity is directly contradictory. Two studies in the 1960s found nulliparity to be associated with poorer outcomes for babies (231, 302). However, three subsequent studies found higher mortality rates in the babies of multiparous women (245, 200, 197). These findings are yet another fine example of how research can leave us none the wiser.

The Canadian Consensus on Breech Management at Term stated that "parity should not influence a decision for planned vaginal birth" (284).

PELVIMETRY

Pelvimetry is the estimation of the size of the pelvis, which is done in an attempt to predict how well the baby will pass through it. The technical name for the problem that pelvimetry is trying to identify is "cephalopelvic disproportion" (or CPD) (sometimes termed fetopelvic disproportion) – essentially a mother's pelvis being too small for the baby's head. An obstetrician is also likely to be interested in the shape of the pelvis. A very straight or flattened sacrum is also thought to cause problems in labour (252).

Pelvimetry can be done clinically (by external examination) or through X-ray or some other form of scanning. Most people talking about the use of pelvimetry are referring to the latter. There is an assumption in some quarters that clinical pelvimetry is "inexact and prone to subjective interpretation" (259), though in fact, studies show a high level of accuracy in up to 77% of cases (106, 220). The problem with clinical pelvimetry is that it requires skill. As one consultant obstetrician put it: "there is often a lack of confidence and competence to do it" (115). X-ray pelvimetry is also prone to technical error so it may be that this "more precise" method of pelvimetry does not increase accuracy dramatically.

Despite the fact that links have been found between X-rays in pregnancy and childhood cancer, X-ray pelvimetry is still being used in the UK. One woman had this experience when she tried to question its safety: "I asked if the X-ray would damage my child and my obstetrician said I needn't worry as it was only a one off and it was so late on in the pregnancy. I still don't know if he was right."

In fact, we cannot be sure of the safety or otherwise of pelvimetry which is normally offered to women carrying breech babies after 36 weeks. The studies which do show links between X-rays and childhood cancer do not clarify whether one X-ray late in pregnancy carries a clear cancer risk. However, since we cannot prove it is safe, and the evidence suggests that it may well not be, the above woman's obstetrician's confidence was misplaced and misleading. In the Netherlands, according to one paper, "owing to the possible harmful effect of ionising radiation on the fetus, X-ray pelvimetry has never been used" (300).

Other methods for pelvimetry are computed tomographic (CT) scanning which still uses X-rays but at a lower dosage (82 mrad as opposed to 500–1100 mrad in conventional X-rays) (53), and magnetic resonance (MR) imaging which uses no X-rays (300). CT scanning seems to be becoming more widely accepted for pelvimetry now (115). However, Guy Thorpe-Beeston, who dismisses X-ray pelvimetry as not of benefit and not recommended, comments: "It can be hard enough to get CT for cancer – whether we should be using it for pelvimetry is questionable." Interestingly, one study found that X-ray pelvimetry produced significantly smaller estimates of one pelvic dimension than MR pelvimetry (318), suggesting that MR pelvimetry may support some trials of labour that X-ray pelvimetry would not. The problem with MR imaging is that it is more expensive and in demand than X-rays. If after reading the rest of this section you do decide you want to go ahead with pelvimetry there is nothing to stop you asking for one of these other pelvimetry techniques, but don't be surprised if agreement is not forthcoming. Rather depressingly, scarcity of resources, rather than the safety of your baby may serve to focus your consultant's mind on whether or not they really need pelvimetry data. One study compared ultrasound measurements of pelvic dimensions with X-ray measurements and found ultrasound to be as reliable as X-ray. There are concerns about the possible dangers of ultrasound (289), but until these are substantiated ultrasound might be a better option than X-rays, and perhaps a more accessible option than CT or MR pelvimetry. Given that many women suspected of carrying a breech will be offered an ultrasound anyway (to confirm presentation and position), this may be a sensible way forward for those interested in pelvimetry.

Misshapen or contracted (i.e. very small) pelvises are far more rare than they used to be. Common causes of contracted pelvises include polio, rickets (287) and childhood malnutrition (16), all of which affect the current childbearing population far less than they ever used to. Other factors that may affect pelvic dimensions that are more relevant to today's women are poor healing of a pelvic injury and a possible link between use of the contraceptive pill in adolescence and a restriction in the growth plates of bone (16). However, the prevalence of problem pelvises is likely to have decreased. The number of women who are denied the opportunity to a trial of labour because of poor pelvic dimensions is difficult to ascertain as figures given in studies generally include any abnormality detected during the pelvimetry. The most significant other abnormality to emerge during pelvimetry is likely to be a hyperextended head (see earlier in this chapter) which accounted for just over half the women excluded from a trial of labour in one study (53). By my own calculation, 13.9% of the sample who underwent pelvimetry in this study were excluded on the grounds of their pelvic dimensions.

On the face of it the logic of pelvimetry seems to be straightforward. Smaller pelvises will be harder for babies to pass through, and the breech baby whose head has not had a chance to mould during labour may perhaps struggle more than its head down counterpart to come through a small pelvis. However, opponents of pelvimetry question the reliability of its findings.

All methods of pelvimetry are likely to have a built in measurement error which underestimates to a varying extent the dimensions of the pelvis. This can occur in techniques such as X-ray pelvimetry if the film is taken at an angle. However, clinical pelvimetry is also problematic because critics argue that the dimensions of the pelvis during labour can differ markedly from those measurable in non-labour conditions. The other problem opponents to pelvimetry cite is that pelvic dimensions are not a fixed entity – due to the muscles interwoven with the pelvis it moves and stretches during labour. Pat Thomas states: "it is impossible to predict how the pelvis will behave and what dimensions it will achieve in labour" (287). It is thus worth bearing in mind that if you have had pelvimetry the measurement you have been given is likely to be the lowest possible dimension of your pelvis.

The use of pelvimetry for head down babies is no longer well respected in most mainstream obstetrics, having been dismissed by Enkin et al. (editors of a well regarded summary of current research and practice in pregnancy and childbirth) thus: "Neither X-ray nor clinical pelvimetry have been shown to predict cephalopelvic disproportion with sufficient accuracy to justify elective caesarean for cephalic presentations" (92). In the same book, these authors state "There is no reason to expect that X-ray pelvimetry should be more accurately predictive of cephalopelvic disproportion for breech than it is for cephalic presentations" (92, p143). However, they go on to say that in breech presentations "it is usual to avoid vaginal delivery when pelvic dimensions are even slightly reduced, in an attempt to ensure exclusion of all potential cases of cephalopelvic disproportion".

Is this caution supported by the research? Cheng and Hannah (49) point out that although X-ray pelvimetry is cited as a selection criteria in the overwhelming majority of the studies they reviewed, there is no good evidence to support that its use influences either perinatal mortality or the rate of successful vaginal delivery. Reports of women who supposedly have pelvises too small to be selected for a trial of labour and then give birth vaginally without any problem hardly help the cause of pelvimetry. This happened to three women in Collea et al.'s study (60) while they were awaiting a date for an elective caesarean.

There are also studies which directly question the value of pelvimetry. One study compared one consultant unit which did not use pelvimetry with two others which used it either some or all of the time (31). The results showed that the unit which did not use pelvimetry had a lower elective caesarean section rate and a higher success rate in trials of labour than either of the other two units. Neonatal outcome was similar for all groups. This reduction in elective caesarean without any increase in emergency caesarean suggests that pelvimetry is not only irrelevant to selecting women for labour safely but also actively harmful in causing unnecessary caesareans.

Two studies examining the outcomes of "undiagnosed" breech babies, or those remaining undiagnosed until labour has started also question the role of pelvimetry. One used clinical rather than X-ray pelvimetry on their 24 undiagnosed breeches (59) and the other had no pelvimetry data on any of their 79 undiagnosed breeches (211). This lack of information appeared to have no impact on outcomes for the babies or on the level of success of the trial of labour. One of these studies commented that the value of pelvimetry in the management of breeches in labour "must be questioned" (211).

There are some studies which claim to support the role of pelvimetry but in fact do not. One study which concludes confidently that "Our findings document that CT pelvimetry is an effective tool in the assessment for vaginal delivery of the singleton term frank breech fetus" merits closer examination (53). What the results actually show is that a selection protocol which included CT pelvimetry produced neonatal outcomes which were comparable for vaginal and caesarean birth, and a relatively low emergency caesarean section rate. Interestingly their low emergency caesarean rate was almost identical to that found on the unit in the previous study which did not use pelvimetry (31) (81% and 79.1% respectively). A study designed in this way simply cannot prove or disprove the value of pelvimetry.

However, there are two studies which suggest that pelvimetry may have a role to play in replacing some emergency caesareans with elective caesareans. For a discussion of the merits or otherwise of this see Chapter 11. One study found that the overall rates of caesarean were similar with and without pelvimetry but that those women who did not have pelvimetry had higher levels of emergency caesarean and higher levels of febrile morbidity (i.e., high temperature), probably due to the emergency caesarean rate. The other study with a similar result is the best designed of all the pelvimetry studies as it is a randomised controlled trial (300). MR pelvimetry was carried out on 235 women who were then randomly assigned to a group where the medical team were given the pelvimetry results, or to a group where they were not. The two groups did not differ significantly in terms of their overall caesarean rates, but once again the group with no pelvimetry information had significantly higher rates of emergency caesarean. They also found that the six babies who were born to women with pelvic abnormalities (who would have been excluded from a trial of labour had their dimensions been known) had lower Apgar scores than those born to women with normal pelvic dimensions. However there were no permanent abnormalities in the babies. It is important to note that in these studies there are no reports of head entrapment (more on this in Chapter 10) – one of the fears advanced by proponents of pelvimetry to justify its use.

One explanation for the higher levels of emergency caesarean section in the group where women were not excluded from a trial of labour for having a small pelvis is that small pelvises may slow up labour. This can cause dystocia or "arrest" of labour leading to a need for an emergency caesarean. Proponents of pelvimetry would argue that small pelvises can be "weeded out" prior to labour to save all concerned the effort of an unsuccessful trial of labour.

According to the data we have, albeit relatively small scale, it seems that all that you may be risking by not having pelvimetry is a higher possibility of an emergency caesarean rather than an elective one. Chapter 11 will help you to weigh up the pros and cons of elective versus emergency caesareans. You may decide that replacing elective with emergency caesarean is in fact a desirable outcome. However, it is worth noting that by not having pelvimetry you may generate anxiety in your medical team, depending on their views on the matter. While this may not be sufficient reason to go ahead with it (particularly not if all you are being offered is X-ray pelvimetry) it is certainly worth checking out your obstetrician's views on the matter. It has been suggested that pelvimetry may be valuable for the commitment to vaginal delivery it engenders when a woman's dimensions are adequate: "MR pelvimetry may select cases accurately, but equally likely is that knowledge that the pelvis is adequate gives clinicians the confidence to allow women an attempt at vaginal breech birth, and to manage these labours without fear of borderline bony disproportion" (308). Wendy Savage's pragmatic approach to pelvimetry is worth noting: "I would probably stop doing it except that I know that all the doctors in training would be so full of anxiety that it hadn't been done!"

The Canadian Consensus on Breech Management points out the lack of support for X-ray pelvimetry and states that it should not be a prerequisite for planned vaginal birth, though would anticipate that pelvic dimensions would be assessed clinically as a matter of routine (284). The FIGO recommendations suggest that whatever method clinicians are most experienced in at any given clinic should be used as there is insufficient evidence to recommend any one method over any other (163).

Whether you agree to pelvimetry or not is up to you. You may decide that there is some logic to it, and that if it makes your medical team more comfortable about your delivery to have done one (though of course it could do the reverse) then it may be worthwhile. However you would be quite justified in leaving pelvimetry to one side. In the words of Pat Thomas: "If your doctor offers you pelvimetry the safest advice is to refuse politely but firmly. It will confer absolutely no benefit to either you or your baby" (287)

AGE AND HEALTH OF THE MOTHER

I am not aware of any research relating to breech birth outcomes and age and health of the mother. The Canadian Consensus on Breech Management at Term stated that the conventional view that "'elderly' gravidas [generally viewed as those women over 35!], especially primigravidas, should best be delivered abdominally is based more on anecdotal and emotional grounds than on scientific evidence". They decided that this convention had come about because of a tendency to see breech presentation with any other risk factor (age is considered a risk factor in the obstetric world) as sufficient grounds for caesarean when in fact this may not be warranted. They concluded that "maternal age alone should not preclude planned vaginal birth". They made a similar case for medical or obstetric complications in the mother (such as mild pre-eclampsia) and said that these should not preclude a trial of labour unless the complication is likely to cause mechanical difficulties at delivery.

SIZE AND MATURITY OF THE BABY

Most studies recommend that an assessment is made of the baby's size using ultrasound to exclude small or large babies. However, most of the published studies on the subject of fetal size estimation (which show large margins of error) exclude breech babies from their sample. This leaves obstetricians working on the assumption that estimates of size for breech babies will be as accurate (or inaccurate!) as for head down babies when this may well not be true.

The only study I have come across comparing weight estimations of breech with head down babies assessed a range of methods for estimating a baby's weight from ultrasound findings and found that almost all had significantly higher levels of error when estimating the size of breech babies than for head down babies. It concluded that in order to be 99% certain that a baby will weigh between 1500g and 3999g, the estimated birthweight needs to be between 2400g and 2900g. This dramatically restricts the range and if put into practice would exclude large numbers of women whose babies were of a perfectly acceptable size. Wendy Savage observed: "you're never sure how big the baby is – all these people go round saying 'it's a big baby, it's an enormous baby' and then out comes this little sprat" (252). There seems to be something more than a little unfair about denying women a trial of labour because medicine has not yet come up with a reliable way of assessing the size of an unborn baby.

What of the evidence on outcomes of big and small babies? The concern for larger babies is that they may start to have a higher risk of head entrapment or other mechanical difficulties in emerging. Different studies have come up with different cut off points above which elective caesarean section is recommended. The range is between 3500g (107) and 4500g (223) though is more normally between 3800 and 4000g. It probably makes sense to be evaluating this information with pelvimetry data if it is available. A baby whose weight is at the upper end of the range with a mother who has pelvic dimensions which are relatively large may be less of a concern than where the mother has small pelvic dimensions and a large baby.

Small babies need to be divided into two camps – babies who are light for their age and babies who are small because they are premature. Some babies are sufficiently "small for dates" to be considered to be suffering from intrauterine growth restriction. Other pregnancy books will tell you more about this but there seems to be little evidence that this in itself is a good reason for caesarean section (287). The evidence on prematurity and breech is discussed in Chapter 8. The area is controversial though there seems to be a prevailing view that caesarean may confer benefit for premature breech babies.

PREVIOUS CAESAREAN SECTION

The rule "once a section, always a section" particularly prevalent in the US, is being increasingly challenged in the obstetric world. The Vaginal Birth After Caesarean (VBAC) campaign has been responsible for rolling back a tide of repeat caesareans which research suggests were unnecessary. However, as is so often the case in breech, things move a little more slowly, and the temptation on the part of the obstetrician seeing a supposed risk factor (previous caesarean) combined with breech is often to opt for elective caesarean. Many selection protocols for vaginal breech birth exclude women from a trial of labour if they have had a previous caesarean section.

The reason for the obstetric establishment's concern about vaginal birth after caesarean is a fear that the strain of contractions on the caesarean scar could cause the uterus to rupture causing severe haemorrhage. However, research suggests that this occurrence is so rare as to be offset by the other adverse outcomes from undergoing elective caesarean section. The exception to this is women who have had a previous classical caesarean section leaving a vertical scar. This is considered at much greater risk of rupturing during labour and as a consequence women with such scars are generally still not permitted to labour. There has also been recent concern about women who have only had one as opposed to two layers of suturing (stitching) to their scar having a higher level of uterine rupture. Finally, concern has also been raised about the use of the drug misoprostol for the induction of labour. A recent American study found that it was associated with 5.6% rupture rate versus only 0.2% rupture rate in women who had not received misoprostol (229). However, even with these provisos, the vast majority of women with a previous caesarean section can labour with a very low risk of scar rupture.

There is little reason to think that the concerns about scar rupture should be any different for a breech. Wendy Savage deals with this issue with characteristic clarity:

People are so illogical – this whole business about adding risk factors together – it depends on what the risk factor is. Why should a breech put any more strain on a scar than a cephalic? "Oh well, the manipulations" they say, "but you don't do any manipulations – you just keep your hands off. (252)

There is one study which specifically addressed this issue in breech and evaluated the outcomes for 47 women who had had one previous caesarean section allocated to a trial of labour group (218). 37 of them achieved a successful vaginal delivery and outcomes for babies in this group were comparable to those born by caesarean. There was one case of uterine rupture resulting in haemorrhage and hysterectomy but this was in a woman giving birth to her tenth child and the authors suggest that this was likely to have been the cause of the problem. Maternal febrile morbidity (a sign of infection, measured by fever) was highly significantly greater in the mothers undergoing caesarean section.

The authors point out: "Caesarean sections are performed to protect the mother or the fetus. Elective repeat caesarean section frequently does not achieve either goal", and conclude:

a selective protocol for management of breech presentation after previous caesarean section seems acceptably safe....It appears that if there is risk associated with allowing a trial of labour, it is small or less than that associated with repeat caesarean section. (218)

AMNIOTIC FLUID VOLUME

This is cited as a selection criteria in some studies (259, 249) but rarely discussed in full. The amniotic fluid volume should be "normal" or "sufficient", though the consequences of it not being are not clear. It is possible that fluid abnormalities simply represent a risk factor which obstetricians are reluctant to combine with breech. In a similar way to the apparent irrelevance of the age of the mother, it could be argued that adding amniotic fluid abnormalities to breech to exclude a woman from an attempt at vaginal delivery also lacks logic.

OTHER PERSPECTIVES ON SELECTION CRITERIA

Women's choice

One study based at a hospital in Hampshire provided a breakdown of its reasons for excluding women from a trial of labour for breech (262). Of the 100 participants, 47 did not have a trial of labour. For 22 of these women, this was their own decision (9 of these women had had a previous caesarean section and opted to have another one although this was not being used as an exclusion criteria in the study). It is likely to become more straightforward for a woman to opt out of a vaginal delivery than opt in, though this depends on the views of her consultant. For more information on negotiating for what you want, see Chapter 13.

Undiagnosed breech

Three studies have looked at the outcomes of undiagnosed breeches, those babies whose breech presentation is picked up only in labour (59, 211, 171). One paper states: "There is particular pressure to deliver the breech diagnosed in labour by caesarean section driven by the fear of inadequate assessment and the belief that the perinatal mortality is worse than if detailed antepartum (pre-labour) screening has been carried out" (211). However, the results from all the studies showed that the babies concerned fared no worse than their ante-natally diagnosed counterparts. One study showed that the undiagnosed breech presentations were almost four times more likely to deliver vaginally (171), although this result was made possible by the very low planned vaginal delivery rate at this unit of 11% (171). These results clearly question the value of extensive ante-natal assessment and selection for breech birth. There was some assessment at the point of diagnosis of the breech position, but this was fairly minimal. As already mentioned in the pelvimetry section, one study used only clinical pelvimetry (59), while another used none (211) with no adverse outcomes. Both of these studies viewed the estimation of fetal weight to be of value, though one used only palpation and not ultrasound to assess weight.

Trial of labour

Some people would argue that the most important selection criteria for vaginal breech birth is a trial of labour. Michel Odent describes his own view of a trial of labour thus:

> The first stage of labour is a test, a trial. This is the time when you decide if vaginal delivery is possible. Its useless to discuss it beforehand. The reason for maternity hospitals is that you can decide to do a caesarean day or night, so why do an elective caesarean section?

He goes on:

> If the first stage of labour is easy, fast, straightforward, without any interference at all it means that probably the vaginal route is safe. If the first stage of labour is long, difficult, does not start well and makes you pessimistic, you do not hesitate, you do a caesarean section. This is my strategy: you do not try to know in advance. (212)

Wendy Savage also supports a trial of labour for breech: "I think you should let women have a go and if the baby's too big it won't come down – it's more a question of when you decide to do the emergency caesarean rather than preventing the woman trying" (252). Mary Cronk agrees: "A breech labour is like any other labour: if it starts spontaneously, if it progresses well, the baby will be born" (70).

The implication seems to be that a trial of labour may be the best selection criteria, regardless of attempts to predict outcome made ante-natally. This view is supported by research showing that the degree of dilation on admission to hospital correlates with successful vaginal delivery (211). The implication of this is that a good progressive labour (suggested by higher levels of dilatation on admission) is likely to lead to a successful vaginal birth. The main risk of pursuing the strategy of using a trial of labour as the main or sole "selection criterion" is a probable increase in emergency rather than elective caesareans. There are both pros and cons to this, which are explored in detail in Chapter 11.

SUMMARY

The only selection criterion upon which agreement is universal is the presence of a hyperextended head which can cause serious injury during a vaginal birth, although the prevalence of this appears to be very low. There is little agreement on a range of other factors including the type of breech position, the number of previous pregnancies, pelvimetry, the age and health of the mother, the size and maturity of the baby, previous caesarean section and amniotic fluid volume. Women also have a role to play in making the decision about whether or not to attempt a vaginal delivery, though in practice it may be easier to opt out rather than opt in.

Some have argued that the best selection criterion is the observation of the first stage: if it progresses well a safe vaginal birth is likely to follow; if it fails to progress caesarean section should be considered.

10
The Management of Vaginal Breech Birth

INTRODUCTION

There is so much controversy on the way to negotiating a vaginal breech birth that you might hope to be in clearer waters when you finally arrive at the subject of the birth itself. Sadly not: the same fierce controversy and contradictions dog the discussion of the optimum management of the birth as characterise the rest of the breech debate. The early part of this chapter discusses the various factors which many people believe may make a difference to the outcome of a vaginal breech birth. One of the key themes that runs through almost all these issues is the contrast between a medically managed, interventionist vaginal breech delivery and a spontaneous "hands off" vaginal breech birth. The terms delivery and birth are used deliberately: in a delivery the woman is seen as having her baby delivered by her obstetrician; in a birth the woman is seen as giving birth to her baby with minimal, if any assistance. The latter part of this chapter describes occurrences and techniques specific to breech birth to give you some idea of what to expect if you are having a vaginal breech labour.

EXPERIENCE OF THE TEAM

It is almost universally recognised that vaginal breech birth requires experienced birth attendants present at the birth. However, experience is often difficult to come by. Part of this relates to the escalating caesarean rate for breech, meaning that increasingly obstetricians emerge from training knowing how to do surgery for a breech but rarely or even never having been present at a vaginal breech birth. In years to come this problem will become increasingly acute as the junior doctors of today become the consultants of tomorrow. At least we are currently in a situation where most consultants, regardless of their opinion on the best way to deliver a breech baby, will have been trained in an era where not all breeches were sectioned. Unfortunately, consultants are not always available on medical wards. Indeed, a recent report on mortalities of breech babies found that a registrar was the most likely practitioner to be involved in a breech delivery (265). In less than a fifth of cases were more senior staff involved, and consultants were informed in only half of the cases before delivery. The report commented: "Inexperience at the time of delivery exacerbated the risk for an already hypoxic [oxygen deprived] baby in some cases."

Discussion of the multi-centre Term Breech Trial (127) in Chapter 8 indicates the difficulty with defining and acquiring experience, given the rarity of breech presentation. It is also important to know "Experience of what?" For many obstetricians, experience comes from breech delivery with all the intervention that is part of the traditional medical approach to breech, an approach which others argue is actively dangerous. This point was made by Harold Henderson as far back as 1955: "It is not the number of breech deliveries that a resident [i.e., junior doctor] handles, but how well he is imbued with the correct technique of handling them" (120a). The "correct technique", of course, is a hotly debated subject, as will become clear during this chapter.

There is far greater potential for anxious or inexperienced birth attendants to cause damage at a breech birth than at a head down one. It would seem that breech labours are fairly anxiety inducing to watch. Caroline Flint said of the second stage of a breech labour when the baby's body has emerged and the head is yet to come out:

It always seems like hours that the baby's hanging there. All contractions can stop. The baby wiggles its arms and its chest heaves and you think "oh my god". (103)

Wendy Savage also describes the anxiety that can arise in the final stages of a breech birth.

When the baby's making these convulsive movements you think "oh this baby's trying to breathe and it's not out" and then people start pulling....If you do pull the breech and the head extends, it's an absolute disaster. You've got to have someone who feels confident. (252)

Not only can anxiety lead to poor management of a breech labour, it can also transmit itself to a woman and her partner, resulting in considerable distress. This slow descent with the fear of the baby's head getting stuck (despite research suggesting that this is a very rare occurrence) is perhaps responsible for one woman's traumatic experience of watching her birth attendants during her labour. "We could tell that people were panicking and at one point after Josh's body was out but his head was still in, the paediatrician covered her face and turned away." Josh's arrival in the world appears to have been fairly normal for a breech birth but this account gives us some insight into the fear that vaginal breech labour can generate.

In relation to a medically managed breech delivery, experience is important to enable the most skilled possible use of medical intervention (such as forceps). For a "hands off" approach to breech, experience is important both to have the confidence not to intervene, and also to judge when intervention is necessary.

The seventh report of the Confidential Enquiry into Stillbirths and Deaths in Infancy concluded that "the most experienced available practitioner needs to be involved and should be present at delivery of a vaginal breech birth". It also recommended "structured simulated training...for all staff who may encounter a vaginal breech delivery" (64).

EPIDURALS

The majority of women who have epidurals find them to be of great benefit in terms of pain relief. However, there is increasing evidence that epidurals are associated with a greater need for intervention, including oxytocin (trade name syntocinon) given to speed labour up, forceps and caesarean section (194). Specifically, there is a threefold increase in the use of oxytocin during labour, a threefold increase in instrumental delivery (i.e., requiring forceps or ventouse) and a significant increase in the length of the second stage of labour (138, 232). The evidence from randomised controlled trials suggests that epidurals are associated with a doubling of the caesarean rate (232, 138, 228, 291, 292, 202). Concern has also been expressed about the way that the drop in blood pressure, common after an epidural, affects the placental exchange, potentially reducing the oxygen supply to the baby (69). Recent interest has been expressed in the "mobile epidural" in which a lower dose of anaesthetic is used (often with an addition of opiates) which enables more movement and some sense of the bearing down reflex. However, studies comparing the two showed no difference in the spontaneous delivery rate and a higher level of side effects with mobile epidurals (associated with the use of opiates in mobile epidurals) (61, 62).

The most recent study of the use of epidurals in breech birth found that "epidural anaesthesia was associated with longer duration of labour, increased need for augmentation of labour with oxytocin infusion and a significantly higher caesarean rate in the second stage of labour" (47). Several of the people I interviewed stated that they would not be happy with an epidural being used in a vaginal breech birth. Mary Cronk states that an epidural has no place in her approach to vaginal breech birth: "If the woman needs an epidural it's a sign that the labour is not progressing well and we should proceed to a caesarean section" (70).

Defenders of the epidural might argue that epidurals are not causing any of the above effects and that caution is needed before jumping to conclusions about cause when in fact all that has been shown is correlation or association. One possible alternative explanation which would account for any findings in studies which are not randomised and simply compare women who requested epidural with those who did not, is that women who ask for epidurals already have dysfunctional labours which affect both their need for an epidural and the subsequent need for greater intervention. A dysfunctional labour could be causing higher levels of pain, which might explain the link. However, there are many people who believe that epidurals are directly causally responsible for the increased need for intervention. Evidence supporting this argument comes from studies showing that allowing the epidural block to wear off for the second stage promotes spontaneous delivery (52), as does the use of a lower dose epidural (51). Most of the studies showing the links between epidural and intervention are randomised controlled trials and therefore not subject to the bias of women with painful labours asking for epidurals more frequently. Women who have agreed to participate in the study will simply have been divided into an "epidural" group and a "no epidural" group and their outcomes compared.

The mechanism for this increased need for intervention is likely to be related to an inhibition of the effectiveness of contractions. Given the importance attached to a good progressive labour in breech (212) this would seem to be a particular problem in breech birth. Of particular concern is the woman's inability to push voluntarily, and the consequent lengthening of the second stage. Various factors facilitate contractions in a natural second stage. Donald Gibb described the Fergusson reflex in which there is a steep rise in contraction intensity at the end of labour, and a natural surge in the body's own oxytocin production (115). Alice Coyle described the way in which the head hitting the G spot in the birth canal produces a fetal ejection reflex (69). Women with epidurals miss out on these experiences.

One woman's experience of a breech birth with an epidural illustrates the problem with pushing:

> Thanks to the big dose of epidural I had no sensation below the waist....The midwife kept an eye on the trace from the electronic monitor to see when my contractions were coming. "Here it comes now! Push! Push harder! Push...push...and push again!" she yelled in my ear, as she had probably yelled in many other ears over the years. Push what? I thought to myself; I couldn't feel a thing. I quite clearly remember thinking "I'd better put on a good show to keep them happy", so I dutifully made a few "uuurgh" noises. (281)

In spite of all this there are many obstetricians who would strongly recommend the use of epidurals in a breech labour as a matter of routine, regardless of whether the woman had asked for it. In a survey of registrars' approach to breech published in 1997, 75% reported using an epidural routinely for breech delivery (261). Why? There appear to be two reasons. One is to try to manage the premature urge to push which can be a feature of breech labours. An epidural weakens a woman's ability to push and so may help her to delay pushing until the cervix is fully dilated. However, a premature urge to push does not appear to be present in all breech labours by any means. It is more likely to be present in footling breeches or premature babies where the presenting part is small. Since epidurals are normally effective within 10–20 minutes of insertion, it should be possible to use them if premature pushing seems to be a problem, rather than in every case.

In *A Guide to Effective Care in Pregnancy and Childbirth*, Enkin et al. comment that routine use of epidurals "to abolish the premature urge to push and reduce the resistance of the pelvic musculature may be reasonable but is lacking evidence" (92). They add that "similar or greater protection might be gained by close communication with and careful instructions to the woman". Many people believe that premature pushing can be managed effectively by panting in the knee–chest position which tips the baby's weight forward off the cervix (see Figure 7.2).

The other reason for routine epidural use in breech seems to be to counteract "the decompression effect" which can occur if the baby's head passes through the birth canal too quickly. In rare cases, the pressure changes which can cause internal bleeding in the baby's skull. However, many midwives and obstetricians will gently slow the progress of the head by supporting the baby's body once it has emerged, and would regard this as quite sufficient to prevent a precipitous delivery. One possible argument which I have not come across being used which may have some logic is to examine the differential effects of an epidural in a woman giving birth to her first baby ("a primip") versus women giving birth to subsequent babies ("a multip"). In a primip, stage two is generally far longer than in a multip. Thus if there is any danger to an unmoulded head, this is more likely to be greater for multips, whose babies will pass through the birth canal more quickly. Donald Gibb points out that "the multip of 3 or 4 deliveries does have overwhelming expulsive powers, and unless she can keep control of these, it can be problematic" (115). Primips' babies on the other hand may take an hour or more to make their slow progress down the birth canal. Although this still involves less moulding to the fetal head than occurs in a head down birth, it is far more than occurs in the few pushes that are often all that is required for the multip to give birth to her baby. Thus it may be that the problems of an epidural are more marked for a primip and the benefits of an epidural may be more apparent for a multip. Unfortunately, numbers would make such a study difficult to carry out.

Wendy Savage points out that when the risks of the decompression effect and premature pushing are explained along with instruction in panting, women can generally control a premature urge to push. However, if the urge to push really cannot be resisted, she argues that epidurals can be useful in these cases (252). She also would not rule out using epidurals for pain relief in a breech labour – a sentiment echoed by Guy Thorpe-Beeston who stated that he did not feel there was sufficient evidence not to use an epidural if the woman needed one for pain and that to deny her one in such circumstances would be a "retrograde step" (293).

The authors of the study showing the increased need for intervention in breech births where epidurals were used make the following comment about the role of epidurals in breech birth:

> Epidural analgesia results in a significant decrease in the uterine contraction intensity during the active phase and in the second stage of labour and may be *inappropriate for vaginal breech delivery if the reduction in maternal expulsive effort leads to an increased incidence of breech extraction or caesarean section.* (47) (italics added)

BREECH EXTRACTION AND ASSISTED BREECH DELIVERY

The next several headings address methods of intervention in the birth of the baby. The distinction between breech extraction and assisted breech delivery should be made clear. Although breech extraction is often widely used to describe a medicalised, interventionist approach to breech birth, its meaning is in fact quite specific. It refers to the intervention in the birth of the baby designed to manage the descent of the baby down the birth canal, sometimes from within the womb. It is likely to involve forceps and significant levels of downward traction to pull the baby out. In current practice it is rarely used other than in the birth of a second twin in the breech position. Assisted breech delivery refers to the use of forceps or manoeuvres to facilitate part of the baby's birth, often just the aftercoming head. In weighing up the pros and cons of assisted breech delivery it is important to be clear about the degree of assistance required. Many who would object to the use of forceps to deliver the aftercoming head would not have a problem with using the Mauriceau Smellie Veit manoeuvre (see below) for example.

FORCEPS

In Mitford's book critiquing "the American way of birth", she introduces her chapter on forceps thus:

In the eighteenth century William Hunter, a leading English accoucheur, declared that "It was a thousand pities forceps were invented. Where they save one, they murder twenty". The same thought, phrased in more circumspect language, was to re-emerge in the medical literature of the 1980s after routine forceps delivery for most births had fallen into disrepute. (198)

If forceps have a somewhat medieval seeming quality to them, its because they have changed very little since the sixteenth century when it is thought that they were first invented. Their invention is fascinating, and may go some way towards explaining why the tool has persisted so long in obstetric practice despite a lack of evidence supporting its value.

Forceps were invented in London, circa 1588, by Peter Chamberlen. Jessica Mitford's description of the early days of forceps is so remarkable it is worth reproducing in full:

The Chamberlen brothers, confusingly both named Peter...travelled round England, charging enormous fees, always payable in advance, for attending births. The forceps were concealed in a richly carved locked casket. The brothers went to amazing lengths to prevent information about their instrument from leaking out. Contrary to the custom of the day, they excluded female family members from the delivery chamber; they blindfolded the labouring woman; and to confound the anxious relatives still further [let alone the poor labouring woman!], they made all sorts of diversionary noises such as ringing loud bells, rattling chains, and banging with hammers during the delivery. (198)

By the eighteenth century, many doctors had arrived at the idea of forceps for difficult deliveries and designs proliferated thereafter.

Historically the invention of forceps seems to have been one of the keys to the entry of men into the world of childbirth and one means they had of distinguishing themselves from midwives. This suggests that forceps have perhaps had a symbolic value to the profession and helps to explain the telling plea contained in an article by some obstetricians in 1963: "The authors title question, 'Midforceps, a vanishing art?' must be answered in the negative, so that it will not vanish and we may remain obstetricians, not midwives!" (74). One obstetrician Mitford interviewed for her book said: "To a man with a set of forceps in his hand, every baby looks as if it needs help being born" (198, p112)

In *A Guide to Effective Care in Pregnancy and Childbirth* Enkin et al. question the use of forceps. They point out that because forceps are effective levers, they risk transmitting pressure to the fetal head, and suggest that this may be especially damaging to a pre-term baby (92). "There is at present no unbiased evidence to suggest that routine use of forceps to deliver the preterm baby confers more benefit than harm."

Michel Odent says that their use of forceps at the French maternity hospital where he was a consultant obstetrician was rendered completely redundant, principally by the use of more upright birthing positions (see below) (213).

Obstetricians react quite strongly when we tell them that forceps have not been used at Pithiviers since 1963 – and that as far as we are concerned, they belong in museums. Such passionate reactions should not be surprising, since forceps are as basic to the practice of modern obstetrics as the supine position; by eliminating both we have, in effect, shaken the very foundations of modern obstetrical practice.

He goes on to caution: "it is unfortunately true that the forceps have yet to be designed that are safe in any hands, and there are only a few hands that can safely and gently use any forceps".

When I met with him, Odent confirmed that he would never use forceps in a breech birth. He explained: "When you know the potential of a woman who is free to be in any posture, when you know the trick of a supported squat at the end, you never think of a forceps delivery" (212).

The independent midwives I spoke to were unanimous in their condemnation of forceps. Mary Cronk states simply that delivery using forceps is "a very dangerous way for a breech baby to be born" (70). Alice Coyle comments: "Most of the injuries to breeches happen because of attendants....Some obstetrician thought it [the use of forceps] was a good idea because he didn't want to wait. Doctors aren't good at waiting" (69). Maggie Banks, also a midwife, makes the point that although the mother is anaesthetised before the use of forceps, the baby is not (16). We have no idea what the experience is for a newborn baby being born with forceps, but one might speculate that it would be fairly traumatic.

Fairly typically in breech birth, practices which have become discredited in head down labours have been slower to be challenged. A survey of registrars in the UK published in 1997 reported that 64% of their sample used forceps to assist delivery (261). Some obstetricians would argue that applying forceps to the "aftercoming head" protects it from pressure. Concern is often expressed about breech babies' unmoulded heads entering the birth canal, compared to head down babies' heads which spend hours being moulded during labour. Since Piper Forceps were designed for breech babies' heads and reported in the literature in 1929, there appears to have been only one study evaluating their use. On the face of it, the 1975 study, entitled "Neonatal mortality of breech deliveries with and without forceps to the aftercoming head" appears to support its conclusion that "forceps should be used in all breech deliveries" (196). The study retrospectively looked at 1423 breech births between 1964 and 1973. It compared those births where forceps had been used with those where they had not. They found significantly higher death rates where forceps were not used when babies weighed between 1000g and 3000g. The authors report that most babies born below a kilo died. The fact that there was no benefit conferred above 3000g they suggest may be due to "the increased physical strength and metabolic reserves of the term infant", but conclude that as fetal weight is difficult to estimate it would be most sensible to apply forceps to all births to be on the safe side.

There are various fundamental flaws to this study which are worth discussing in some depth as I am not aware of this having been done elsewhere. Firstly, the authors report that forceps use increased over time from one third of breech births to almost two thirds at the end of the study. It is possible that improvements in other areas such as neonatal care during the period of the study were in fact responsible for the decrease in deaths, but the fact that forceps use increased over the same period enabled forceps to artificially take the credit. The study also reports no details of morbidity which is unfortunate as damage to mother and baby as a result of forceps use are of particular concern.

Another major problem with these results is that on the face of it, one may assume that what is being compared is forceps assisted breech birth and spontaneous breech birth. However, when one studies the methodology in detail, it emerges that the non-forceps group includes "spontaneous, assisted or breech extraction". The proportions of each type of delivery are not specified. Thus what is actually being compared is forceps on the one hand with various types of breech births on the other, including those where the baby is likely to have been pulled out manually. The risks of pulling a breech baby are discussed elsewhere in this chapter in the "hands off the breech" section, but is generally thought to be dangerous. It may well be that forceps confer benefit over other methods of breech extraction or assisted breech delivery, but this study simply cannot answer the question of whether a forceps delivery confers benefit over spontaneous breech delivery. The best, and to my knowledge only, comparison of interventionist methods of delivery versus spontaneous breech birth is described in the next section about the Bracht manoeuvre.

Thus we are left with no evidence to support the routine use of forceps. Wendy Savage suggests that they can be used to bring the head down more quickly if there is fetal distress (252). But in general, it would seem that you are on strong ground to challenge your consultant if he/she recommends the routine use of forceps and you do not feel comfortable with this.

THE BRACHT MANOEUVRE

The Bracht manoeuvre sounds more technical than it is in reality. It is a method for assisting the birth of the baby using the birth attendant's hands as gently as possible. Proponents of the Bracht manoeuvre contrast it with classical procedures. Classical procedures are described as involving more active obstetric intervention, often forceps, and are characterised by downward traction in which the baby is essentially pulled out to try to hasten the delivery. Authors of a paper on the Bracht manoeuvre point out:

The aim and object in the deliveries of vertex [head down] presentations are to assist, to supplement and, if necessary, to enforce that mechanism which represents the basis of spontaneous deliveries. For reasons which are not entirely clear, no such principle has guided the obstetrical world in its approach to the problem of breech deliveries. (230)

The Bracht manoeuvre appears to try to mimic the mechanics of spontaneous delivery in the all fours position. The diagrams illustrating its use show a woman lying on her back and the baby's body being lifted gently towards the mother's pubic bone, much as would occur naturally through gravity in an all fours position. The instructions for its use state "The force applied in this procedure should be equivalent to the force of gravity." Although one may be left wondering if there is in fact any value of the procedure over and above good old gravity, the value of the paper is that it provides some data comparing this method of largely spontaneous delivery with more traditional methods of breech delivery.

The 1953 paper on the Bracht manoeuvre I looked at is in essence a meta-analysis before such a concept was invented: essentially a bringing together of several studies to create a large sample (2987 breech deliveries, of which the Bracht manouvre was attempted in 1719 cases) (230). It is made clear that using the Bracht manoeuvre is not exclusive – it can coexist with classical procedures which can be employed if the obstetrician feels they are required. Recourse to classical procedure was required in 168 of the 1719 cases. All the studies were European or South American. The manoeuvre seems to have been almost universally ignored in the UK and the US, where classical procedures have dominated. The average mortality rate for all the studies employing the Bracht manoeuvre was 1.39% with five of the studies (with sample sizes of up to 206) reporting a 0% mortality rate. The authors contrast this with mortality rates for breech babies reported in the British and American literature of 4.4% and 4.98%. While these rates are higher than is the case now for historical reasons (e.g., less good neonatal intensive care), the difference does indeed suggest that classical obstetric management of breech delivery may have been contributing to the mortality rate. The authors go on to look at two studies in particular which give data from their institutions pre- and post-introduction of the Bracht manoeuvre. Prior to this introduction, solely classical manoeuvres were used. The change of a mortality rate of 5.1% with classical manoeuvres to 1.4% with the Bracht manoeuvre with classical procedures where necessary was statistically significant. Although the comparison between two time periods could perhaps be explained by other factors, it does offer further possible support for the Bracht manouvre.

A slightly more recent study from Holland in 1971 found a mortality rate of 1.55% in 163 cases of breech birth, the majority (78.5%) managed with the Bracht manoeuvre (130). This is particularly impressive as the selection protocol was minimal, excluding only estimated low birthweight babies (below 2500g), cases of placenta praevia, second twins and intrauterine deaths. The authors comment of the Bracht method:

Active participation of the woman in the expulsion is of great importance. Primary administration of anaesthetics [such as epidurals which prevent the woman's participation] seems, in our opinion, very objectionable in breech presentation. (130)

The authors of the review paper make a powerful case for spontaneous delivery to be at least tried, and intervention on the part of the obstetrician to be minimised:

The chances of surviving the delivery for babies presenting by the breech decrease with the degree and time of interference. The more manipulation is performed and the earlier this manipulation is instituted, the greater is the fetal mortality and morbidity, to say nothing of maternal injuries....If this is correct, the efforts of the obstetrician should be directed toward cutting down the time and extent of manipulation, to avoid the necessity of its employment...The art of waiting is a difficult one, and not many obstetricians have either the courage or the patience to sit idly by while the breech delivers spontaneously; this becomes even more difficult if the impatient obstetrician has a century of tradition as well as the words and writings of all contemporary teachers behind him. (130)

They conclude that the adoption of the Bracht manoeuvre in the US should lead to a considerable reduction in the breech mortality rate and that further rigorous research was required. This appears never to have happened and the Bracht manoeuvre is barely mentioned in the British and American literature.

The research on the Bracht manoeuvre represents the closest we have to an evaluation of spontaneous breech birth. Logic would suggest that a technique of birthing a breech baby which used gravity (such as using an upright position) may confer even greater benefit than the Bracht manoeuvre which is merely attempting to mimic gravity.

THE BURNS-MARSHALL METHOD

The Burns-Marshall method for delivering the aftercoming head is not dissimilar to the Bracht manoeuvre and is far more widely recognised in the UK and US. In fact it intervenes later in the birth process in that the baby is allowed to emerge spontaneously until the shoulder blade appears. The ankles are grasped and swung upwards (creating an upward force similar to the Bracht manoeuvre until both arms are free). The body is then allowed to hang until the head descends into the pelvis and the hair line shows. This is the Burns-Marshall method; the attendant is then free to choose their approach to the remainder of the birth.

In a survey of registrars in the UK, 20% reported using the Burns-Marshall method (261).

THE MAURICEAU SMELLIE VEIT MANOEUVRE

This extraordinarily named manoeuvre is commonly used to help the birth of the head. The baby's legs are either side of the attendant's arm. The attendant places their first and third finger on the baby's cheek bones and their second in the baby's mouth to help flex the baby's head (or keep it flexed). Wendy Savage recommends using the cheekbones only and avoiding the mouth as she suggests there is a risk of dislocating the jaw (252). The attendant then hooks two fingers of the other hand over each shoulder from the back and pulls the baby down (16). A French study recently evaluated the use of the manoeuvre in 103 breech babies and found no difference in the complication level between this sample and the general neonatal population (94a). In a survey of registrars in the UK published in 1997, 64% reported using the Mauriceau Smellie Veit manoeuvre (261).

Although Maggie Banks describes this as a manoeuvre to use when the baby's head is extended, it appears to be frequently used by many of the people I spoke to as a matter of course (115, 212, 252).

THE LOVSET MANOEUVRE

The Lovset manoeuvre allows the attendant to release raised or, more rarely, nuchal arms (i.e., arms that become stuck above the baby's head). Once the baby is born to the umbillicus (the navel), the baby is grasped, carefully ensuring that no pressure is applied to the baby's kidneys. The baby is pulled down and rotated, and the attendants fingers are then inserted into the vagina to bring down the arm (16).

Maggie Banks comments that nuchal arms are usually created by the hasty attendant pulling on the baby's body, and also suggests that necessity for its use can be reduced by having women in upright positions. She gives the example of Mary Cooper, an American home birth midwife who attended 89 breech births with babies weighing up to 4650g, all in upright positions. Only one baby needed minimal assistance to have an arm brought down. I have not come across data on the prevalence of nuchal arms so it is difficult to establish the impact of upright positions.

"HANDS OFF THE BREECH"

It is for good reason that the mantra of many highly experienced midwives and obstetricians is "Hands off the breech", often with a postscript of "sit on them if necessary". Caroline Flint describes her approach to stage two thus: "My bottom line is to try never to do anything" (103). Wendy Savage agrees: "You just encourage her to push, you don't have to do very much really. The most important thing to say to a registrar is 'don't touch it'" (252).

The temptation to pull is a common but potentially lethal response to anxiety. Flint (105) cites Margaret Myles' textbook for midwives, which lists the dangers to the baby during a breech birth which all relate to intervention on the part of the attendant. These include damage to the brachial plexus caused by twisting the baby's neck and causing Erb's paralysis (of the upper arm), ruptured liver caused by grasping the abdomen, damage to the adrenals caused by grasping the baby at kidney level, crushing the spinal cord or fracturing the neck by bending the body backwards over the symphysis pubis while delivering the head. This makes terrifying reading, but the important implication is that they are all preventable.

More recently an obstetrician described the problems of pulling thus: "Pulling on the baby greatly increases the risks of deflexion of the fetal head and extension of the fetal arms, both of which may greatly increase the difficulty of the delivery and the risks of fetal trauma" (249). Caroline Flint, in her review of the literature on potential trauma suffered by the baby during vaginal breech birth, says: "according to most of the literature the greatest danger to the baby seems to be the trauma caused by the person delivering the baby being over anxious and too rough in their delivery techniques" (105).

Gregory White, in his *Emergency Childbirth Manual*, emphasises the importance of "hands off the breech" because "more breech babies die of injuries received at the hands of their would-be rescuers than die of smothering [oxygen deprivation]" (cited in 105).

Mary Cronk tells the story of a medical colleague at Queen Charlotte's Hospital many years ago who described his own approach to breech consisting of getting a pint of beer, sitting and facing the corner and waiting for the baby to be born (70). Although there is likely to have been a little exaggeration for comic effect in his account (though perhaps he really did – who knows?), the point about non-intervention is clearly made. Mary Cronk has followed this hands off approach herself and advises not even touching the woman's anus during birth to wipe away faeces so as not to cause any muscle spasm and interfere with the process.

Jane Evans emphasises the importance of understanding the limitations of a "hands off" approach. "Its no good saying 'hands off the breech' until the baby's dead. You have to know the mechanisms for helping a baby in the very rare event of a problem" (94).

"HANDS ON THE BREECH"

The only exception to the hands off the breech rule in the natural breech birth arena is found in a video of six breech births produced by Ina May Gaskin and her midwives of the Farm in the United States. Ina May Gaskin is a highly experienced self-taught midwife and author of the book *Spiritual Midwifery* (113). People continue to flock to the Farm where she still practises, to have natural births often when they have become disillusioned or unhappy with what mainstream obstetrics has to offer. The video makes remarkable viewing (details of how to get hold of a copy can be found in the Useful Contacts section). At every breech birth there appear to be multiple female birth attendants surrounding the labouring woman and her partner. A midwife carefully holds the baby soon after its bottom emerges and gently wiggles it out with a side to side motion. To any believers in the "hands off the breech" approach, it initially makes fairly excruciating viewing. However, Ina May appears to know what she is doing; the introduction to the video contains a section on the dangers of grasping so one assumes that the precise location of the grasp is carefully considered. Two of the six births involve babies with nuchal arms (raised and stuck above the head) which she handles calmly and confidently.

Interestingly almost all the labours and births shown are in a semi-seated position. It is perhaps the failure to use gravity in these births which has necessitated the interventionist approach, and it seems possible that the combination of the semi-reclining position and hands on approach may have made the occurrence of nuchal arms more likely. However, the outcome data available, although the sample is small, suggest that the intervention is sufficiently gentle and skilled not to compromise the baby. Of the 60 vaginal breech births attempted at the Farm, all were successful and none required caesarean section (113).

In spite of the contrast in management styles, the midwives at the Farm have key characteristics in common with advocates of "hands off the breech" in their approach to the woman. They have a profound belief in the woman's ability to have a go at giving birth to her baby, and they work to reduce fear. This sets them apart from a more traditional medical interventionist approach.

POSITIONS FOR LABOUR

Lithotomy, supine and dorsal positions

Lithotomy is the position where a woman lies flat on her back with her legs in stirrups to hold them wide apart. Supine is simply lying flat on the back without the feet up. In a dorsal position the shoulders and chest are raised but the woman is still essentially lying down; this is sometimes referred to as a semi-seated position. The lithotomy position can have a distressing, inhuman quality to it, quite apart from problems with its mechanical efficiency discussed below. One woman's vivid account of her experience of lithotomy during a breech labour is a powerful one:

I heard a jingling noise and realised it was my legs, suspended by the ankles in chains from metal posts, desperately and involuntarily trying to come together. After a lifetime of socialisation which teaches us to hide our genitals, to be so exposed in front of strangers is a horrible experience. (281)

Tradition has it that the lithotomy position started in seventeenth century France when Louis XIV had his mistress endure labour in this position so that he could have a better view of the birth of his child from his hiding place behind a curtain (213). It was around this time that men started to become involved in childbirth and forceps were invented. The lithotomy position follows logically on from the use of forceps – it provides optimum accessibility and visibility for the forceps user.

Guy Thorpe-Beeston defends the lithotomy position for stage two of a breech labour thus: "very often we do have to assist the aftercoming head and be in a position to do so relatively quickly". He also points out that research on the relative merits of one position for breech over another is not available and concludes "In this day and age, I don't think that evidence is going to come to light" (293). Interestingly it has been suggested that the lithotomy position where a section of the bed is removed so that the woman is no longer resting on her coccyx is mechanically preferable to supine or dorsal positions where the weight on the coccyx constrains the space for the baby.

Enkin et al., in *A Guide to Effective Care in Pregnancy and Childbirth*, draw attention to "Forms of care likely to be ineffective or harmful" (92). They state that there is clear evidence that the use of both a supine position and lithotomy position is ineffectual or harmful. Lying down may lengthen the second stage of labour, reduce the incidence of normal births, increase abnormal fetal heart rate patterns and reduce umbilical cord blood pH values (a sign of lack of oxygen). Tellingly they add: "Although some birth attendants report that upright positions caused them inconvenience, there has been a consistently positive response from the women who have used an upright position for birth" (92). Wendy Savage points out that many women feel ill on their back and that around 6% suffer from supine hypotension syndrome (where the blood pressure drops as a result of lying down). She believes that even those who do not experience acute levels of hypotension are likely to suffer from some degree of reduced blood flow to the placenta.

Michel Odent strongly advocates the use of a supported squatting position in breech birth and comments: "We would never risk a breech delivery with the mother in a dorsal or semi-seated position" (213). The reasons for this criticism are twofold. The first is that there is good evidence that lying down reduces the dimensions of the pelvic capacity. Estimates of the increase in pelvic capacity from supine to squatting have been made at as much as 1cm and at 28% in different studies (105). These differences are significant; they would be sufficient to exclude a woman from a trial delivery if a protocol using pelvimetry were employed and her dimensions were on the borderline. With any birth, maximising the pelvic dimensions is important but this would seem to be of particular importance with a breech birth where anything that contributes to the baby's smooth and easy passage is to be striven for. The other key criticism of lithotomy, supine and dorsal positions is that they fail to use the help of gravity. Gravity helps bring the baby down and keep the head flexed (105). In White's *Emergency Childbirth Manual* he states: "In order to add the weight of the baby to the forces helping delivery, the mother should be assisted to a position on her hands and knees" (cited in 105).

Wendy Savage commented on her own reaction when she first advocated a standing position instead of lithotomy: "It was just so easy compared with having the mother with her legs in the air!" Interestingly, Mary Cronk argues that bringing down a nuchal arm is far easier with a woman not in lithotomy as there is so much more space in the hollow of the sacrum. In lithotomy the attendant needs to squeeze their hand in between the weight of the baby and bed.

In her 1989 paper, Caroline Flint concludes with a plea:

I would encourage obstetricians to examine the way breech babies are being delivered and to ask themselves whether this way [a supported squat] might not be more rational – taking cognizance of the effect of maternal posture on pelvic diameters and the effects of gravity. (105)

Active birth positions

Supported squat or standing breech birth

These two terms seem to be used in the breech literature to describe the same position. The woman normally stands holding on to her partner or birth assistant. Gina Lowden, who writes from personal experience on the subject of breech, says:

For a supported squat a strong, supportive husband whose neck you can hang round is really useful, or perhaps a midwife on either side with your arms across their shoulders. Student midwives may be very willing to oblige if it means they can participate in a natural breech delivery as these are so rare. Another possibility may be to hang from your hands from the lithotomy stirrups. Some initiative and imagination could be helpful on this one!! (175)

Michel Odent explains his reasons for recommending the supported squat position for breech birth thus: "it is the most mechanically efficient. It reduces the likelihood of our having to pull the baby out, and is the best way to minimise the delay between the delivery of the baby's umbilicus and the baby's head" (213). He points out that this position can be rapidly transferred into from an all fours position if extra gravity is needed at the point of birth by lifting the woman from behind, supporting her under her armpits. She can then hang in a squatting position. He emphasises the importance of an interested partner not bending over to have a look at the emerging baby as this radically reduces the efficiency of the position. Bending forward would also put considerably more strain on the partner's back. Yehudi Gordon comments on the power of an upright position and contrasts it to an all fours position: "All fours is much less powerful in the second stage than squatting – it makes sense. You wouldn't sit on the loo on all fours, you'd be sitting or squatting" (123).

However, this position is not without its critics, even amongst those who support active birth. Mary Cronk, has expressed her concerns about an upright position for breech birth. She questions whether so much gravity is needed at this stage, saying that it is better for the baby to move gently down. She also expresses concerns about the safety of the baby:

It seems to me that if the woman is vertical there may be some traction on the cord/placenta from gravity just after the birth and in the absence of a contraction....when the woman is standing, the birth can be too swift and the placenta can separate too quickly; assisted too much by gravity, it can arrive almost on top of the baby's head. (70)

She goes on to say "I do not have any evidence to support this theory but I feel that until I have evidence to refute it, I should not encourage women to give birth to breeches in a vertical position." Jane Evans, another independent midwife, also stated she was not happy with women standing to give birth to a breech baby (94) (though both Mary and Jane point out that in their experience women rarely seem to take up a standing position of their own accord). Wendy Savage agreed that premature separation of the placenta could be a concern and had attended one woman where this had occurred (252). However others argue that this is not the cause of positioning but merely a rare and chance occurrence in breech labours. Guy Thorpe-Beeston argues that this premature separation of the placenta does not seem to happen in standing births for head down babies so it is no more likely to for breeches (293). While this may be true, clearly premature separation of the placenta has potentially more serious consequences for breech babies because there is longer before the baby's head emerges.

An audit was carried out at the Chelsea and Westminster Hospital in London on just over 20 cases of standing breeches (293). Three of the total sample suffered poor outcomes – an alarmingly high percentage. It is difficult to draw conclusions from such a small study, and the fact that it has not been published leaves us in the dark about selection and labour management protocols, and also what went wrong in the three cases and whether this was likely to be attributable to the mode of delivery. It is also unclear as to whether it was the position that was responsible or some other factor. Guy Thorpe-Beeston suggests that it may have been due to a lack of experience in managing a standing breech birth (293).

All fours position

Mary Cronk and Jane Evans favour an all fours position (70, 94). When the mother is on her hands and knees the uterus is horizontal and tipped forward, thus not putting the strain on the placenta which she highlights as potentially problematic for a more upright position. She also suggests that women are more likely to assume an all fours position naturally if not directed otherwise. It also provides a more flexible use of gravity. If more gravity is needed the woman can kneel up and lift her body up; if things are moving too fast she can drop into a knee–chest position. Caroline Flint, during her description of a standing breech birth, suggests that the woman should lean forward as the head is emerging to bring her trunk into a horizontal position to help release the nose and mouth, and points out that this enables a combination of posture and gravity to do what many obstetricians would use a manoeuvre to effect (103).

A word of caution

Jane Evans cautions that active birth should not be about adhering to a prescribed gravity efficient position no matter how the woman feels. "Active birth means actively listening to what your body is saying because it's right" (94). She gives an example of a woman who, in spite of her intention to labour on all fours, felt far more comfortable lying down throughout the labour, until immediately before the birth when she briefly assumed an all fours position to push the baby out. It emerged that the baby had been sitting on its cord and that the woman's instinct to be horizontal had been the most appropriate way of keeping pressure off it.

Perhaps the key to finding your way through these conflicting views on positions is keeping an open mind and being flexible, adjusting your position according to the needs of the situation and what feels right at the time.

CREATING THE RIGHT CONDITIONS FOR VAGINAL BREECH BIRTH

Michel Odent said of his approach to breech birth: "The point is not to deliver the breech baby; it is to create the conditions where the woman can give birth to the baby" (212). Of particular importance in his approach is enabling full and uninhibited progression towards "the fetus ejection reflex" often misconstrued as a "second stage" as a result of a cultural misunderstanding of birth physiology (214). He quotes one father's comment about his wife's birth as follows:

I find it strange that when we talk with our friends about childbirth, they constantly refer to a first stage and a second stage. When my wife gave birth she had no second stage. She had a sort of sudden reflex and soon after the baby was born. (214)

Odent describes the fetus ejection reflex as powerful and irresistable contractions during which there is no room for voluntary movements, but cautions that

all events that are dependent on the release of oxytocin (particularly childbirth, intercourse and lactation) are highly influenced by environmental factors....It does not occur if there is a birth attendant who behaves like a "coach" or an observer, or a helper or a guide or a "support person". It can be inhibited by vaginal exams, eye to eye contact, or by the imposition of a change of environment. It does not occur if the intellect of the labouring woman is stimulated by rational language ("now you are at complete dilatation you must push"). It does not occur if the room is not warm enough or if there are bright lights. (212)

He suggests that the true role of the midwife is to protect an environment that makes the ejection reflex possible, reconciling the labouring woman's need for privacy and need to feel secure. He argues that in breech birth it is "more imperative than ever" not to deviate from these circumstances (212). Although his views of the role of fathers and other support people in the labour room have sparked some controversy, many people in the active birth world would take a similar view of the sensitivity of the labouring woman to her environment and the importance of getting this right for the individual woman.

The irony for women carrying breech babies is sadly that it may be far harder for them to create the circumstances that are ideal for a vaginal breech birth, than for women carrying a head down baby. Their anxiety is likely to have been heightened by their medical team and others' attitudes to vaginal breech birth. Instead of being attended exclusively by one or two midwives, women are likely to have a doctor, if not several, present. Michel Odent comments: "It's as if with a breech you are expecting something a little more difficult than the average and you make it still more difficult artificially – it should be the opposite" (212).

THE USE OF OXYTOCIN/SYNTOCINON FOR SPEEDING LABOUR UP

The use of oxytocin for speeding labour up (augmentation) is hotly debated for breech babies. It is considered in cases of "hypotonic dysfunctional labour" – cases where labour is not progressing normally. There are many people who would argue that a breech labour that is not progressing well is an indication for caesarean section (115), and that to speed it up with oxytocin could cause fetal distress and/or driving the baby's body through the pelvis and its head getting stuck.

Some studies argue against its use (34, 216, 37, 296, 117, 267) whereas others suggest that it causes no harm (245, 60, 142, 118, 207). A survey published in 1988 of American perinatal obstetricians found a split with 43% of respondents saying they would augment a breech labour and 57% saying they would not (11). A similar survey of Canadian obstetricians found that 78–83% of obstetricians (depending on the type of breech) would augment labour (224).

Michel Odent is clear on the issue, saying: "I would never use syntocinon because it would stop the first stage from being a test. It would be artificially too easy. We have to evaluate the physiological potential of this woman in labour" (212). Yehudi Gordon is even clearer: "No way – if you need to boost contractions, god knows what's going to happen to the head" (123). Mary Cronk is equally adamant about the dangers of augmentation stating: "Syntocinon has no place in breech birth – if contractions are not progressing the woman's body is telling you something and you should listen" (70). She criticises the use of syntocinon to achieve a vaginal delivery no matter what the cost to mother or baby. All of the above would recommend proceeding to a caesarean section in the event of contractions failing to progress.

Wendy Savage, on the other hand, argues strongly for the use of syntocinon just as it would be used in a head down labour, based on the fact that in a term baby the diameter of the hips is the same as that of the head.

If you accept that the hips'll go through, there shouldn't be any problem with the head so long as you don't pull on the breech and extend the head. I don't believe that you can drive the baby through if it's too big to go through the pelvis. You've got to have adequate contractions to see if the woman's going to deliver. (252)

Donald Gibb agrees stating that he would use oxytocin if contractions are poor (115).

INDUCTION

There are similar debates over the use of oxytocin to induce labour as there are for its use to speed labour up. Wendy Savage argues in the same vein as above that she cannot see the logic of not inducing. One study looked at induction in breech by comparing the induction of 46 women with breech babies to the induction of 46 women with head down babies. They also compared these groups with 23 breech babies undergoing a trial of labour and 23 born by elective caesarean section. There were no differences between the groups and 52.2% of the women in the induced breech group delivered vaginally. The authors conclude that induced vaginal delivery appears to be "safe for both fetus and mother". The numbers in this study are small, however. In the survey of Canadian obstetricians on breech management, 69–78% of respondents (depending on the type of breech) said they would induce a woman with a breech presentation (224).

If you are late and threatened with caesarean section if you do not spontaneously go into labour or do not wish to be induced if it's offered, you may want to try some of the following natural methods of starting your labour.

Nipple or breast stimulation is now well accepted as a natural method of induction (or augmentation) (218), though there are those who suggest that the contractions this produces may not be akin to true labour contractions and if prolonged may present a threat to the baby's oxygen levels (305). This method is believed to work through triggering the body to release natural oxytocin. Another natural method of induction is sexual intercourse. This is thought to help in various ways. The man's sperm contains oxytocin, and the woman's orgasm both releases oxytocin and triggers muscular contractions that can trigger labour. Penile pressure on the cervix also causes the release of oxytocin. A trial comparing breast stimulation and no prohibition of sexual intercourse with no stimulation and a prohibition of sexual intercourse from 39 weeks of pregnancy found that fewer women in the first group had late babies (92).

Acupuncture claims to have methods of encouraging labour to start, as does reflexology, so it may be worth consulting practitioners of these alternative therapies. Many people take the classic herbal approach to labour induction as raspberry leaf, taken either as tablets or tea. However, raspberry leaf is thought primarily to tone the uterus, making contractions more efficient, rather than stimulating labour. Nicky Wesson, herbalist and author of several books on pregnancy, recommends the homeopathic remedy caullophyllum 30c to be taken every hour or half hour to be continued once labour has started to ensure that its effects do not wear off. If this does not work, the more potent dose of 200 can be dissolved in a glass of warm water and drunk until a third remains, topped up with water and then drunk till a third remains, etc. This can also be used when membranes have ruptured but there are no contractions (313).

THE USE OF WATER IN VAGINAL BREECH LABOUR AND BIRTH

Many obstetricians will not consider a breech water birth. They suggest that being in a birthing pool would not enable them to monitor and control the labour and delivery properly. There is also the problem that water births are generally not considered for "abnormal" labours, so finding anyone with any experience of a breech water birth is likely to be challenging.

However, there are those who believe that water birth is as much an option for breech as it is for head down births (16). Indeed, one could argue that a water birth could directly help some specific problems in breech birth. There is a belief that contact with the air stimulates babies to breathe (82). One concern with breech babies is that if there is much time elapsing between the birth of the baby's body and its head, the baby may try to breathe when it cannot yet access air with its nose and mouth. (This may explain Mary Cronk's observation that breech babies are often slow to breathe (70) – perhaps there is an inbuilt mechanism delaying breathing to maximise the chances of the head having emerged when the baby takes its first breath.) Presumably if the baby is born into water (which will be maintained at body temperature during a water birth) this will help by delaying the first breath until the baby is fully born. The other advantage of a water birth is the pain relief it can provide for a mother. Many women may choose not to opt for epidural during a breech birth and the pain relieving properties of water may be particularly valuable. It is important to recognise the distinction between labouring and giving birth in water, and if you make it clear that you intend to use water only for pain relief and will get out when the moment of birth is approaching, your birth attendants should be open to this.

Caroline Flint pointed out that giving birth to a breech baby in water reduces the benefits of gravity (103). Michel Odent expressed a concern that using water in stage one of a breech labour would make it artificially easy and therefore not a true test of the woman's potential (212). Annie Francis, independent midwife, suggested that water can often slow labour down, particularly if the pool is entered too early. She cautioned that in a breech labour, progress can slow for other reasons which may not be picked up if the woman is in water. It is interesting that none of the people I spoke to were particularly comfortable with the idea of a breech labour in water. However there is a centre in Ostend in Belgium who specialise in water birth and have produced a video of breech births in water and a booklet about their work (82). They do place some qualifications on who may be suitable for a water breech birth, stating that they tend to select multiparous women (i.e., with one or more previous pregnancies) and frank breech babies. However, the following quotation suggests that they may be willing to "have a go" in other situations given the ease of resorting to alternative delivery methods if necessary:

We do admit that nulliparous women seldom have a breech delivery underwater, this due to the frequent demand for epidural analgesia and/or necessity to have a perfusion of oxytocin. If one has successfully delivered one child, breech delivery is perfectly possible underwater. All manoeuvres are perfectly possible underwater, if things go really wrong you can get out of the bathtub and have a "classic" breech delivery, or if all goes wrong, caesarean section. (81)

The Belgian centre's contact details can be found in the Useful Contacts section. Maggie Banks has photographs of a breech labour conducted in water in her book (16).

FETAL MONITORING

There are debates about the benefits of different types of monitoring and the reader is referred to Pat Thomas' book *Every Woman's Birth Rights* (287) or to the Midirs leaflet on *Fetal Heart Rate Monitoring in Labour* (195) (see the Useful Contacts section for details on how to contact Midirs).

There are those who strongly recommend the use of electronic fetal monitoring (EFM) in breech labours: "Electronic fetal heart rate monitoring is essential in the management of labour in breech presentation", argues one paper (259). One concern that has been expressed in research on EFM is that it increases the caesarean rate without improving outcomes for babies by identifying distress where in fact none is present. It is recommended that fetal scalp blood sampling – a technique for sampling and testing the baby's blood to provide information about levels of distress – is used to check the results from EFM (280). In breech babies, the fetal "scalp" monitor can be fitted to the baby's bottom and blood samples taken from there (175). It could be argued that, for these circumstances at least, the breech baby has judged its position well. If offered the choice of having blood sampled from my scalp or my bottom, I know which I'd opt for every time!

Maggie Banks argues that intermittent monitoring, which has the great benefit of not restricting the woman's movement, is adequate during a breech labour (16).

CORD PROLAPSE

Cord prolapse refers to the umbilical cord dropping into the vagina. This is most likely to happen when the waters break and carry the cord with them. When the presenting part is not firmly engaged in the cervix, the cord may slip through the cervix and into the vagina. Cord prolapse occurs on average in 3.7% (172) to 7% (259) of breech labours, compared to only 0.3% of head down labours (65). The higher incidence in breech is because of the less good fit between bottom and/or feet and cervix compared to head and cervix. Rates of cord prolapse increase with prematurity, multiparity (numbers of previous pregnancies) and most significantly in flexed breeches, especially footling (259). In fact, the occurrence of cord prolapse in extended or frank breeches is 0.4%, essentially the same as for a head down baby (259). The incidence goes up to 5–10% for complete breeches, and to 10–25% for footling breeches (259). For more information on cord prolapse see "Position of the baby" in Chapter 9.

The majority of babies survive cord prolapse and cord prolapse with a breech is less risky with a breech than it is with a head down baby (175). There are many instances of cord prolapse where the baby appears to suffer no adverse effect (119, 324). In the Term Breech Trial, 14 babies suffered cord prolapse, and none had an adverse outcome (127). In a breech baby the legs may shield the cord from compression, and the pressure on the cord may not be as great (and therefore not as life threatening) as it would be with a head pressing on it. However, there are trials where mortality rates following cord prolapse are higher than 30% (49). The variability in outcome may relate to how closely the labour is monitored and what protocols are in place for managing cord prolapse. Donald Gibb has stated that "cord prolapse in supervised care doesn't kill a baby – poor management of a cord prolapse does" (115).

How cord prolapse is managed

If cord prolapse occurs early enough in labour, caesarean section will be recommended as quickly as possible. You may find yourself surrounded by panic stricken staff and are likely to be put under general anaesthetic, though if there are no other signs of fetal distress, the urgency may not be so great (175). If the cord prolapses during the second stage and delivery is imminent, the vaginal delivery may well be continued though often with an increased urgency.

What to do if your cord prolapses

You should adopt the knee–chest position (see Figure 7.2) with your face near the floor and your bottom in the air. This tips the baby's weight away from the cervix and should reduce the pressure on the cord (though obviously it is not a good position to assume if it has been decided that going for a rapid birth is the best option when an upright position would be preferable). If you are at home, medical help should be sought urgently (probably in the form of an ambulance), and unless birth is imminent or the hospital is too far away, hospitalisation arranged immediately.

Donald Gibb, a consultant obstetrician, has suggested the following practical advice for a woman who finds herself without professional help and aware that her cord is in her vagina:

The cord goes into spasm if it hits cold air. If your cord slips out of your vagina, replace it as quickly as possible. Even if the cord is simply sitting in your vagina, your baby will stand a better chance of survival if the cord is not exposed to air. (115)

A midwife may insert a finger into the vagina to lift the presenting part off the cord.

CORD COMPRESSION

Cord compression occurs when the umbilical cord is squashed between the baby's head and the mother's pelvic bones resulting in a reduction of blood flow and therefore oxygen to the unborn baby (16). Cord compression is a concern in breech birth because, unlike in head down birth where the head is born ahead of the umbilical cord, a certain amount of cord compression by the head once it enters the birth canal is inevitable. There is debate about the implications of cord compression. Yehudi Gordon, who for much of his career favoured vaginal delivery, now prefers elective caesarean section because of cord compression. He says: "You can always get cord compression – you can never fully predict it" (123). However, he does admit that the small number of cases which changed his approach to breech birth where cord compression was a problem were not typical and were perhaps not optimally managed.

Others disagree, not so much that cord compression occurs, but about its significance for the baby. Donald Gibb states:

There is no question that you get more cord compression with breeches. But babies were designed to tolerate cord compression – cephalic babies get it as well. Cord compression doesn't present an acute threat to the life of the baby. (115)

Caroline Flint also suggests that cord compression is of no great concern:

I never worry that much about cord compression. I mean, look at cords – they're so thick and springy. Trying to get a cord clamp on them is sometimes murder! They can be pressed, but they can only be seriously compressed by the head and the head shouldn't be there for very long anyway. It's not something that terribly fusses me. (103)

John Stevenson, a home birth doctor living in Australia, argues that cord compression is not responsible for the baby's heart rate slowing in the second stage of labour. However, the implication of what he says is similar – when the baby starts to show signs of oxygen deprivation birth needs to be completed within a relatively short space of time.

At this point of rumping (or crowning) it is worth noting the time, because this is when the oxygen is cut off, not for the mistaken reason given in textbooks that baby's head compresses the cord against mother's bony pelvis, but for the obvious and realistic reason that the uterus contracts and shrinks down behind the descending baby, and in doing so it cuts off the maternal blood supply to the placenta. This cutting off of baby's oxygen is often signalled by a sudden slowing of baby's heart rate to well below 100, not because of anoxia [oxygen deprivation] (it happens well before baby starts going blue) but an automatic reflex slowing in order to conserve the oxygen in baby's system. (The same slowing is often noticed with crowning in a vertex birth; it is of no significance then, because the birth will be completed within a minute or two.) But in a breech, you need to contemplate that within 30 minutes at the very most, or within 15 to 20 minutes at the least, baby will be in trouble with anoxia. But as the body descends, you can usually count on completing the birth within the very safe limit of 10 minutes. (276)

In an article entitled "The 'stress' of being born", the authors compare the slowing of the heart rate to conserve oxygen to what happens to animals when submerging themselves in water for a dive (163a). Wendy Savage points out: "Babies are designed to be born – they've got their anaerobic respiration. They can last for five minutes whereas grown ups can only last for two without oxygen to the brain" (252).

HEAD ENTRAPMENT

Scorza reports three factors as potentially responsible for difficulty in the birth of the aftercoming head:

1. head entrapment due to an incompletely dilated cervix
2. hyperextension of the fetal head
3. unrecognised disproportion between the size of the fetal head and the pelvic dimensions (259).

The second two are discussed elsewhere – hyperextension is an indication for caesarean and should be picked up on ultrasound before labour has started (see Chapter 9). The baby's head becoming extended during delivery is a rare and avoidable complication (259). It is most likely to occur if the baby is pulled down rather than being left to descend of its own accord. Scorza suggests that moderate suprapubic pressure can be used to keep the baby's head flexed if necessary (259). Fetopelvic disproportion is discussed in Chapter 9 under "Pelvimetry". Evidence seems to suggest that when disproportion creates a problem in breech birth it is simply in increasing emergency caesarean section, probably due to labour not progressing.

Head entrapment as a result of an incompletely dilated cervix is more common in premature, growth restricted or footling breech babies. An incompletely dilated cervix can in fact probably account for a phenomenon known as "clamping" of the cervix, which is sometimes mentioned in the non-academic literature on breech. Proponents of the idea of cervical clamping assume that having fully dilated, the cervix then clamps on the baby's neck and prevents the head from passing through. However, it seems that clamping is more likely to be a misdiagnosis of complete dilation, which illustrates the dangers of premature pushing. Scorza gives the following example to illustrate the ease with which an incompletely dilated cervix can be missed:

A typical situation in which this dreaded complication occurs is when a mother in preterm labour arrives with bulging membranes and a nonfrank breech. The cervix often is mistakenly assumed to be fully dilated, and the patient feels the urge to bear down. When the membranes rupture, the fetus is delivered up to the head, and the cervix is clamped around the unfortunate fetus's neck. Relief at this point can only be provided by complete uterine relaxation, Durhrssen's incisions [a series of cuts in the cervix viewed as obsolete in obstetric practice except for this situation] or abdominal rescue [by caesarean section]. (259)

In spite of the alarm surrounding the subject, cases of head entrapment in the literature often have surprisingly favourable outcomes (241). Wendy Savage questions the prevalence of head entrapment as an issue:

People are so worried about the head getting stuck. In my experience the head doesn't get stuck unless the cervix isn't fully dilated. Maybe I've just been lucky, but I've never had a head get stuck. Actually when you ask people, very few have had that experience. Before ultrasound, heads did get stuck if there was a minor degree of hydrocephaly [enlarged head] that couldn't be felt abdominally. There's a sort of folk memory. With ultrasound, so you get rid of the hydro-cephalics, and leaving the breech alone, so you don't pull down and extend the head, I don't think heads do get stuck. (252)

EPISIOTOMY

Episiotomy, rather like forceps, has seen a dramatic reduction in use over the last decade or two from being routine practice some years ago. Sheila Kitzinger and the work of the National Childbirth Trust helped to challenge its routine use:

Women often say that they feel they are "sitting on thorns" [after an episiotomy]. Such acute pain in an already tender area may affect the way a woman holds and handles her baby and interfere with the easy start of breast-feeding. The NCT (National Childbirth Trust) showed that women who had torn are more likely to be able to hold their babies comfortably than those who have had episiotomies. (156)

Some people argue that an episiotomy can help with delivery of the head of a breech baby though I have not come across any justification for the argument that it should be routine in breech. It has been suggested that women with no previous children are more likely to need an episiotomy (252), but this can be judged during the second stage of labour. Interestingly the independent midwives I spoke to had mixed views of this with one saying she tended to use episiotomy more frequently in breech birth and another saying she rarely found it necessary.

CATHETERISATION

Catheterisation, or the use of a thin tube to empty the bladder, is worth considering where labour is not progressing. A full bladder can hold up the presenting part and women can lose sensation and fail to realise it is full. Because of the higher expectation of a need for caesarean section in breech labours it is particularly important to bear in mind the possibility of this being necessary. It is possible that birth attendants may jump to the conclusion that your labour is not progressing for other reasons without having catheterised you first to make sure. Charlotte's birth story illustrates this perfectly. Charlotte was told that vaginal birth for her breech baby would not be a problem because she was tall and her baby was small.

I progressed slowly but surely. I resisted the suggestions for an epidural, saying I would wait and see. I got to 8–9cm but then got stuck and was given a further four hours before a caesarean. Every time a contraction came I was desperate not to push but it was very hard. The four hours came and went and I was desperate and exhausted and signed the consent form for a caesarean. A catheter was put into my bladder and released heaps of liquid (probably at least 1 pint if not more)! Suddenly the contractions went wham! And I was in transition, shivering etc. The midwife had disappeared to arrange for a single room for me for after the caesarean! The registrar came back in, saw the situation and said we would try vaginally as he could see that things were suddenly progressing, saying it would be general anaesthetic if things went wrong. It took an hour and a half and I delivered in theatre. I was high on gas and air and was given a huge episiotomy. My legs were in stirrups but I was too exhausted to care. Isobel came out bottom first, legs and all. Once she started coming, there was no stopping her and the registrar got poo and wee over his face she was so keen!

MECONIUM

Meconium is the black tarry bowel motions that the baby experiences in the first few days after birth. Its appearance during a normal head down birth is often taken as a sign of fetal distress. However, during a breech labour, the contractions apply force to the baby's tummy and bowel and can force the bowel to empty (175). The presence of meconium only becomes significant when heart tones are abnormal (16).

Maggie Banks recommends the rupturing of membranes if they are still intact when the baby's bottom is on the perineum (i.e. just about to emerge from the vagina). This ensures that any meconium in the waters will drain out and keeps it away from the baby's head as it is born (16).

LENGTH OF LABOUR

Gina Lowden comments that labour with a breech presenting part may be longer and more difficult because the baby's bottom does not "fit" the cervix as closely as the head. The force of the contractions bearing down on the cervix which make it dilate is therefore not as strong or efficient (175). This is presumably more likely to be an issue for flexed breeches, particularly footlings where the presenting part is less likely to fit as snugly.

There is no particular reason to think that a long stage two is more likely or more of a problem in a breech birth. However, keeping a close eye (or ear) on the baby's heart rate is important. Donald Gibb states: "It's not long second stages that damage babies, its long second stages with abnormal fetal heart rate patterns" (115).

IMMEDIATELY AFTER THE BIRTH

It seems to be common for breech babies to be slower to breathe (71, 105) immediately after being born, though many breathe without help and have high Apgar scores. It is important that both staff and parents are prepared for this possibility, so that the necessary resuscitation equipment is on hand and there is not too much shock and fear generated by the situation. Beatrice, whose daughter Teri was born in a natural vaginal birth which went smoothly describes the following scenario immediately after the birth:

> It was a breeze for me but a shock for her and the first few minutes were horrendous. I didn't really see her before she was whisked away, but my husband did and thought she was dead. She was completely blue, floppy and not breathing. Her Apgar score, I found out later was 2. Despite initial predictions that she would need a night in the baby unit, she made a very quick recovery and didn't need any further help after ten minutes or so....I wish I had been warned and we had all been better prepared for the possibility of her needing respiratory help.

Alice Coyle, independent midwife, cautions that it is crucial not to cut the cord too soon with a breech baby for precisely this reason. The cord may still have valuable oxygen coming through it which may help the baby to adapt to its first minutes outside the womb (69). However, this may be difficult to negotiate if your birth attendants need to resuscitate the baby at some distance from where you are – umbilical cords will not reach as far as a resuscitaire. It is worth discussing this issue beforehand.

SUMMARY

The management of a vaginal breech birth is immensely controversial and particularly striking for the coexistence of starkly opposing views. Some argue that epidurals and forceps are essential to promoting safe vaginal delivery while others argue that this is actively harmful. The little evidence we have seems to suggest that less interventionist approaches permitting more spontaneous breech births are associated with better outcomes. The various manoeuvres used to assist in breech babies – Bracht, Mauriceau Smellie Veit, Lovset, and Burns-Marshall are described. Active birth positions which maximise pelvic dimensions and utilise gravity are described, as are the benefits of a "hands off the breech" approach and the importance of creating the right conditions for a vaginal breech birth. The "hands on" approach of the American midwife Ina May Gaskin is briefly described. The use of drugs for starting off and speeding up labour is also discussed, with some believing this is a dangerous intervention in breech birth and others arguing it is entirely legitimate. The evidence on this issue is mixed. Alternative approaches to inducing labour (including intercourse and nipple stimulation) are described. Conflicting views on the use of water in a vaginal breech labour and/or birth are given. The options of continuous or intermittent fetal monitoring during labour are raised.

The problems and management of cord prolapse, cord compression and head entrapment are discussed and some DIY suggestions are offered for dealing with cord prolapse if it occurs. The phenomenon of head entrapment is described, which in term breech babies with well managed labours seems to be rare. Outcomes from head entrapment seem to be generally favourable. The issues of episiotomy, catheterisation, meconium staining and length of labour are also discussed specifically in relation to breech. The tendency of breech babies to be slower to start breathing immediately after the birth is also mentioned.

The ideas discussed in this chapter may help you to formulate a birth plan, discussed in more detail in Chapter 13.

11
Emergency Caesarean Section After a Trial of Labour: Not the Worst of Both Worlds?

Emergency caesarean section was a scary idea – to me it conjured up images of panicking doctors shouting at one another as they wheeled me down to theatre at breakneck speed, preparing to put me under general anaesthetic as they did so. I remember the dilemma of thinking "Here I am trying to give birth to my baby vaginally, and I may end up not even being conscious when he arrives in the world – at least an elective caesarean section with an epidural would ensure I witness the birth." Although some emergency caesarean sections are indeed emergencies, the majority in breech birth are far from it. The literature often uses the term "intrapartum" caesarean section, meaning "during labour", which is a more accurate and less anxiety inducing way of describing it. The terms "unplanned" or "unbooked" have also been suggested (69). The most common reason for an emergency section being performed in breech is "failure to progress". In one study this accounted for 81% of intrapartum caesarean sections for breech (30). In such situations the decision to operate may be arrived at over many hours. Even emergency section performed for fetal distress may not be as dramatic as it sounds; unless the distress is severe and acute there may be no great rush while all involved weigh up the relative merits of allowing labour to continue or proceeding to a caesarean section.

THE RELATIVE DANGERS OF EMERGENCY VERSUS ELECTIVE CAESAREAN SECTION

When outcomes of emergency versus elective caesarean sections have been compared, emergency caesareans always seem to have higher levels of complications for mothers – both in terms of morbidity and mortality. Guy Thorpe-Beeston points out that emergency operations in other medical fields such as appendix removal or ectopic pregnancy are also riskier (293). However, the extent of the increased risk of an emergency section is a matter of considerable debate. Some estimates are as high as 6.5 to 1 or 5.1 to 1 for the risk of maternal morbidity following emergency over elective caesarean section (210, 221). Bingham and Lilford, in a complex paper on the implications of these risks for the management of breech delivery, explored the question of how best to protect women's health (30). They challenged the assumption that striving for vaginal delivery of breech babies protected women's health. They argued that if approximately 20% of trials of labour ended up in an emergency section with the consequent increase in risk for women over elective section, then ultimately a policy of elective caesarean section for all women may produce fewer complications and maternal deaths. This is an interesting and potentially persuasive idea. However, three years later, the same authors with two others published another paper re-examining the relative risk of emergency versus caesarean section. They point out that the risks associated with emergency section are not the same as the risks attributable to, or caused by it. For example, it is not the fault of an emergency caesarean section if an acute medical condition which has necessitated the urgent operation midway through labour later kills the mother. Their analysis looked solely at complications such as post-partum haemorrhage, infection, pulmonary embolism and anaesthetic complications which could clearly be said to be caused by the operation itself. They compared these factors in emergency and elective section and found a relative risk of 2 to 1, far lower than suggested in other papers. They cite the relative risk of death following all caesarean sections as being between sevenfold and thirteenfold that of vaginal delivery and conclude that the argument for elective surgery to protect women's health no longer holds water.

Sadly this U-turn in policy recommendation seems not to have fully permeated the obstetric profession, as this woman's experience at a London Teaching Hospital in 1998 illustrates: "I was told that I should have an elective caesarean section because the risk of complications from an emergency section was five times greater" (i.e., 5 to 1).

WHY ARE EMERGENCY CAESAREAN SECTIONS MORE RISKY?

Nobody really knows the answer to this, but some possible hypotheses can be advanced. The first is that true emergency caesareans, i.e. those which are done in a hurry to remove a baby who is in severe danger, are bound to be more prone to mishap than an elective operation. There has been no analysis done of emergency sections carried out in this way compared to sections performed in no particular hurry because labour is not progressing. Several of the people I spoke to testified to the fact that caesarean for a breech labour was invariably needed for a lack of activity rather than an emergency. In the words of Mary Cronk: "There isn't a panic – this baby ain't going nowhere – there's plenty of time to calmly proceed to a section" (70). If the majority of caesareans for breeches are done for the non-urgent condition of failure to progress, one could perhaps argue that emergency caesareans for breech may be less damaging for the mother. However, no studies have been done on emergency caesarean specifically in breech so this must remain purely speculative. Guy Thorpe-Beeston cautions that an urgent section could simply be required if a woman who was planning a caesarean section was admitted at full dilation, so suggests that even without a medical emergency, the policy of waiting for labour to start could necessitate a true emergency section (293). However, in such a scenario it may be appropriate to re-examine the basis for proceeding to a caesarean, given that the indications from such a progressive labour could be to go ahead with a vaginal birth.

A second possibility is that elective caesareans are generally scheduled within the working day. More emergency sections are done in the middle of the night with staff who may be fatigued and who are likely to be more junior than those present at a section during the day.

Guy Thorpe-Beeston also points out a third possibility which is that women may have been less prepared for an emergency section and may have eaten or drunk beforehand, risking anaesthetic complications if a general anaesthetic is required. However, if the section was planned, starvation could be observed during labour assuming that things did not progress too rapidly. It has also been pointed out that anaesthetic complications can be managed in other medical settings (e.g., emergency surgery on road traffic accident victims who will not have fasted beforehand) and so this should not present a significant problem in obstetrics (159).

THE POSSIBLE ADVANTAGES FOR BABIES
OF EXPERIENCING LABOUR

Although there is little research in this area, people are increasingly starting to suggest that labour, even if it does not end in vaginal birth, may be beneficial for babies. There are two main areas of suggested benefit. The first is in the timing of birth. The problem with elective caesarean section is that doctors are keen to schedule it a good safe distance before your due date – often between ten days and two weeks. This is for various reasons, but mainly it seems so that an emergency or intrapartum section, with all its supposed inconvenience and risk can be avoided. However the problem is that at 38 weeks (the time elective sections are normally booked in) the baby may be only just maturing. If there has been an error in estimating the due date and the baby is in fact younger than 38 weeks old at birth there may be some consequences of this prematurity, such as breathing difficulties. Some people argue that what determines the onset of labour is a poorly understood mechanism, but that it seems possible that the baby is somehow triggering the birth process at a point when it is ready to be born. Babies born by elective caesarean section are deprived of reaching this state of readiness.

The second benefit proposed of the experience of labour is documented in a fascinating paper called "The 'stress' of being born". The authors introduce their paper thus:

At first thought, being born would seem to be a terrible and dangerous ordeal. The human fetus is squeezed through the birth canal for several hours during which time the head sustains considerable pressure and the infant is intermittently deprived of oxygen (by the compression of the placenta and the umbilical cord during uterine contractions)....In addition, during the strains of birth – particularly hypoxia (oxygen deprivation) and pressure on the head – the fetus produces unusually high levels of the "stress" hormones adrenaline and noradrenaline [part of a group of hormones known as catecholamines] – higher than in such severely taxed adults as a woman giving birth or a person having a heart attack. (163a)

Indeed, such a conception of birth may be one reason why increasing numbers of women favour caesarean. There is a sense that in some way to protect their babies from this ordeal it is the kinder and easier option. The authors continue:

In spite of surface appearances, the stresses of a normal delivery are usually not harmful. Evidence collected by us and others during the past two decades indicates that the fetus is well equipped to withstand stress…; indeed it is the catecholamines that afford much of the protection from such adverse conditions as hypoxia (oxygen deprivation). Moreover, it is actually important to undergo the events eliciting the production of stress hormones. The resulting surge of hormones prepares the infant to survive outside the womb. It clears the lungs and changes their physiological characteristics to promote normal breathing, mobilises readily usable fuel to nourish cells, ensures that a rich supply of blood goes to the heart and brain and may even promote attachment between mother and child. (163a)

The fact that this surge of hormones appears to protect the baby not just from the birth process but also prepares it for life outside the womb led the authors to a discussion of "the possible over use of caesarean section". They report research showing that babies delivered by elective caesarean section without labour had low catecholamine levels, whereas those delivered by emergency surgery (after labour had begun) had a surge only slightly lower than that of vaginally delivered infants. Their own research suggested that at two hours following birth, babies delivered vaginally had significantly better lung function than those delivered by elective caesarean section. They suggest the following link between this finding and breathing difficulties following elective section:

Infants delivered by elective caesarean section are known to be predisposed to breathing difficulties. Two major factors are inadequate absorption of lung liquid at birth, which gives the lungs a wet look, and inadequate production of surfactant: a soaplike substance that decreases surface tension in the alveoli of the lung (where oxygen and carbon dioxide are exchanged) and allows them to remain open. The absorption of lung liquid and the release of adequate surfactant both appear to depend on the sustained increase in plasma catecholamines in the hours immediately before the birth. (163a)

They conclude:

Taken together, the weight of the evidence indicates that the elevation of "stress hormones" in the normally delivered newborn reflects not only a response to acute stress but also an attempt by the body to enhance the chances for survival at birth. Such findings suggest that infants delivered by elective caesarean section before the mother begins labour may be at some disadvantage.

One way to overcome the disadvantage might be to administer catecholamine like drugs to surgically delivered newborns, but this approach has yet to be proved safe and effective. In the meantime some obstetricians, particularly in the U.S. are now attempting to give the infant the benefit of a catecholamine surge by delaying surgical delivery – when they can – until the mother has experienced at least the early stages of labour. (163a)

Although this paper does not focus on breech babies, it turns on its head the notion that "elective caesarean is best for baby". It would seem that, depending on your reading of the research, the best outcomes for babies may be achieved through vaginal delivery or emergency caesarean section, with elective delivery trailing in last place. Elective section does have benefits for mothers over emergency section, but given the dramatic difference between outcomes for mothers between caesarean and vaginal births, it could be argued that the mothers' best interests are served by a trial of labour. One is left with the possibility that the only person for whom elective caesarean section is best may be the obstetrician.

POSSIBLE BENEFITS FOR THE MOTHER'S NEXT LABOUR FROM EXPERIENCING SOME LABOUR

There have also been suggestions that there may be benefits for any subsequent birth in experiencing some labour. These benefits are thought to be twofold. Firstly, it has been suggested that a caesarean wound on a womb that has already thinned somewhat in labour may heal more strongly, and consequently be less likely to rupture in a subsequent labour. Secondly, it may also carry advantages in terms of the length of a subsequent labour. Second labours are often thought to be signifi- cantly quicker and more progressive than first labours but an elective caesarean section first time around will mean that your second labour is more like a first one. Experiencing some labour first time around may help to reduce the length of a subsequent labour. This applies even if you have not had any dilation and your cervix has simply started to efface (become thinner) (69). In a climate where vaginal birth after caesarean is termed "trial of scar" and where obstetricians carefully monitor and limit the length of labour for fear of placing too much strain on the scar, all the help you can get in speeding up a second labour is worth having. If you are not planning to have any more children this point is clearly less relevant to you.

THE EMOTIONAL IMPACT OF AN EMERGENCY CAESAREAN

The emotional impact of caesarean is described elsewhere in many excellent books and websites on the subject (eg,109, 321a). The specific challenge of adjusting to an emergency caesarean relates to altered expectations and a possible sense of failure. Indeed the term "failed trial of labour" which is used routinely in medical circles may contribute to the feeling that somehow the mother just did not have what it took to succeed. Feelings of inadequacy and depression can follow. There may also be the added trauma of fetal distress occurring and anxiety about how it may affect the baby.

The main difference in a breech labour compared to labour with a head down baby is the higher rate of emergency caesarean. Assuming you have been fully informed, you should have been told that any trial of vaginal breech labour has anything between a 1 in 5 to more than a 1 in 2 chance of ending in caesarean. This gives you a greater chance to prepare for the possibility of a caesarean. While preparation won't take away the understandable hope that caesarean won't be necessary and disappointment if it is, it may mitigate it somewhat. Some women may draw considerable comfort from a feeling that at least they tried, and are also reassured by knowing that the surgery they experienced was necessary.

Everyone has their own individual reactions to circumstances such as this. However, it is important to challenge the idea that women undergoing emergency caesarean are always distressed by the experience and wish they had opted for an elective section.

SUMMARY

The term emergency caesarean is something of a misnomer, particularly in breech. With 81% of "emergency" caesareans in breech being caused by failure to progress, the process of taking the decision to operate is likely to be a lengthy and leisurely one. There are figures suggesting that emergency caesareans are riskier for mothers, but initial estimates of 5 or 6 to 1 (emergency to elective) have since been revised to 2 to 1. The reasons for this may include some emergency caesareans being carried out in a hurry or at night and consequently with less care. There is good evidence that any labour occurring before an emergency caesarean helps the baby to breathe better in the first hours of life. Some people also think that going into labour enables the baby to signal when it is ready to be born and that this may have far reaching consequences. It has also been suggested that experiencing some labour may facilitate subsequent vaginal birth. Emotionally an emergency caesarean section can be difficult to adjust to. However, at least the higher rate of caesarean in breech gives you a chance to prepare for the possibility of such an outcome. Some people feel comforted by the knowledge that they tried and that the caesarean they had was the only option.

Part Four

Making a Decision About the Birth and Negotiating for What You Want

12
Making Your Decision About the Birth

INTRODUCTION

You may have already made your decision about the way you are going to have your breech baby, in which case this chapter may be of little use or relevance to you. However, even if you are booked in for an elective caesarean, you may wish to consider the arguments for emergency over elective caesarean. Some of the options described in this chapter are not freely or easily available, and are taken up by a tiny minority of women carrying breech babies. But it seems important for you to at least know about these various possibilities, even if it is to reject them as not right for you or not practical in your own circumstances. I am sure that there are many arguments that I've omitted and would not pretend that this is a conclusive guide to decision making about breech birth. But I hope it provides a basis for your own decision making, even if it is only to start you off down what can be a long and at times agonising road.

WHY YOU MIGHT WANT TO HAVE A VAGINAL BIRTH

If you find yourself wanting a vaginal birth, having a baby presenting by the breech may force you to justify that want/need/instinct in a way that head down babies do not. Michel Odent, playing devil's advocate, asked me "Why make the effort to give birth by the vaginal route when it is so easy to do an elective caesarean section?" (212). The reasons for your choice can be divided into two groups – those related to the mother and those related to the baby.

Reasons for aiming for vaginal birth relating to the mother

At a very basic practical level, vaginal birth leaves you dramatically healthier than caesarean birth. It should not be forgotten that a caesarean is major abdominal surgery. In addition to the far greater risk of short term infection and the higher risk of maternal death, there are also the longer term risks caused by the presence of the scar which can complicate future pregnancies and births. Caesarean birth is often promoted as the convenient way to give birth. However, apart from being able to select the time of an elective caesarean, the reverse is true in terms of health and recovery time. This can be particularly problematic if you have an older child or children who also require your attention in the weeks after the birth. You may be told not to pick up your older child for weeks or even months after a caesarean. This can be a serious problem for anyone with a child aged under 3, necessitating fairly intensive support post-operatively.

Guy Thorpe-Beeston points out that some consideration should be given to the number of children a woman is likely to have. Generally three caesarean sections is regarded as the maximum (293) (though apparently, Bobby Kennedy's wife, Ethel, had at least nine! (252)).

In an emotional sense, a positive experience of birth can have far reaching consequences. Fran, who gave birth to her first (and second) breech baby vaginally, said:

"I think that the post-natal period with all its ups and downs was enhanced and made more manageable by my birth experience. I've read somewhere that to experience labour and birth in a positive and empowering way creates mothers (and fathers) who have increased confidence in their ability to parent well."

Reasons for aiming for vaginal birth relating to the baby

Chapter 11 details the evidence on the beneficial "stress" of being born. In summary, research suggests that, contrary to being traumatic for the baby, the process of natural birth stimulates a hormonal reaction in the baby which improves its chances of survival after birth, principally by making breathing easier in the first few hours of life. There have also been suggestions that this process may give a kick start to the baby's immune system.

Michel Odent is adamant that "being born is not just to enter the world and be alive at birth. Probably the way that we are born has long term effects on our lives" and cites mother–infant bonding which we know can be affected by birth experience as an example of the significant consequences of the way we are born (212).

These benefits for the baby have to be weighed against the possible risks of a vaginal breech delivery, as described in Chapter 8. However, my own conclusion from reviewing the evidence is that in most cases of breech presentation it is difficult to be sure about the safest method for the baby to be born.

Three of the five obstetricians I spoke to regarded vaginal breech birth as a legitimate and safe option (Wendy Savage, Donald Gibb and Michel Odent), as did all the independent midwives (though dependent on the way it is managed (see Chapter 10). Although they are not a representative sample, their views are nonetheless valid. All three shared the view that women should be allowed to "have a go" and that this was the best test for establishing whether breech birth was viable (see Chapter 10 for a more detailed discussion of this). Michel Odent was more concerned about the circumstances in which this trial of labour takes place and has suggested that emergency caesarean may be preferable if the situation is not ideal (see below) (212). On the other hand, Wendy Savage was so adamant that a trial of labour was the right course of action for the vast majority of women carrying breech babies that she objects to suggestions that women should have a choice about whether or not to have an elective caesarean. She states categorically: "I don't think they should have the choice...I don't think the evidence is there to put it that way." She goes on:

Breech birth is no more unpredictable than any labour. I know there are people who say you should section every woman. I think that is a silly route to go down. Now we've got ultrasound we should be much better at letting women have a go. We can always bail out – it's not as if we're in the middle of Africa when you're 600 miles from the nearest hospital – so we should be able to just let women get on with it. (252)

One important issue to bear in mind if you are opting for a trial of labour is to regard it as just that. In most studies a majority of women succeed in giving birth vaginally, but the rates of women who go on to have emergency caesareans often approach, and sometimes exceed 50%. Many people regard positive thinking as being an important component in vaginal birth, but you have the challenge of managing this alongside being open to the very real possibility of a caesarean being necessary. Both Yehudi Gordon and Donald Gibb draw attention to the dangers of becoming overinvested in a vaginal birth and this potentially overriding decisions about the safety of the baby. Guy Thorpe-Beeston emphasises the importance of holding both the exciting possibility of a successful vaginal birth and the real possibility of a caesarean in mind at once:

If she succeeds, that would be great and she would feel fantastic about it, but she needs to go into it understanding that there's round about a 50% risk of caesarean section at the end of the day. If she succeeds she'll be up and about much more quickly, carrying around a huge sense of achievement which you can't put a number on. (293)

Reasons you may want to aim for an active vaginal birth

The reasons why many people believe active breech birth to be safer than vaginal breech birth with forceps and epidural are discussed in detail in Chapter 10. These include the greater use of gravity and bigger dimensions of the pelvic outlet when in an active birth position. Concern is also expressed about the lengthening of the second stage of labour with an epidural and the potential for damage to the baby with the use of forceps. This needs to be weighed against medical concerns about a birth which is too quick or where the head is not protected from the pressure of rapidly descending through the birth canal. However, this can be managed by an experienced birth attendant with a change of position if necessary. There may also be psychological benefits to feeling more actively involved in the birth process.

Risks of vaginal birth

Unlike the risks of caesarean section (see below), the risks of vaginal birth are much harder to quantify because of the debate about whether any negative outcomes are caused by factors inherent in the process of vaginal breech birth, or due to poor delivery technique. As Caroline Flint states:

On looking through the literature one learns that although obviously there must be increased danger of the baby's head being trapped at delivery when the cervix is not fully dilated, according to most of the literature the greatest danger seems to be the trauma caused by the person delivering the baby being over anxious and too rough in their delivery techniques. (105)

Ralph Wright, writing in 1959, known as the first advocate of routine caesarean section for all breech babies, lists the following risks of a vaginal breech birth (320):

1. compression of the umbilical cord
2. the baby's body slipping through an inadequately dilated cervix
3. trauma to the unmoulded fetal head
4. difficulty in determining the presence of cephalopelvic disproportion (where the woman's pelvis is smaller than the baby's head).

All the issues covered here are addressed in more detail in Chapter 10 (with the exception of cephalopelvic disproportion, discussed in the "Pelvimetry" section of Chapter 9).

One study suggested that vaginal breech delivery had a five times greater risk of obstetric brachial plexus (nerves in the neck and armpit) palsy (paralysis) than head first deliveries, some but not all of which may resolve naturally over time (114). Premature babies have a higher risk of sustaining such injuries (205).

Risks of caesarean section

The risks of vaginal birth largely relate to the outcome of the baby. However, the risks of caesarean section concern both mother and baby. The risk of the mother dying following elective caesarean section with no emergency present was 2.84 times greater than if she had a vaginal birth (125) in one analysis. This figure was calculated from the UK Confidential Enquiries into Maternal Deaths in 1998. Other studies suggest the higher levels of a three to thirteen times greater increase in maternal mortality of caesarean versus vaginal delivery (258, 148, 173) when emergency and elective sections are included.

Other risks include the morbidity associated with any major abdominal surgical procedure (such as anaesthesic accidents, damage to blood vessels, accidental extension of the uterine incision, damage to urinary, bladder and other organs) (307). Guy Thorpe-Beeston says he would explain to any woman considering a caesarean the risks of haemorrhage, anaemia, infection and thrombosis, all of which can happen with a vaginal delivery but are more common with a caesarean (293). 20% of women develop fever after caesarean (306), although in a recent study there was no difference in the morbidity of women with caesarean and vaginal births at six weeks follow-up, apart from a longer stay in hospital in the caesarean group (127). In another study, however, women who had their babies delivered by caesarean section were twice as likely to be readmitted to hospital in the first three months following their caesarean as women who had had spontaneous vaginal births. Research generally shows women undergoing caesarean section spend significantly longer in hospital than women having a vaginal birth (306), and recovery times on discharge are slower with women having to wait six weeks before they can drive and also having to be cautious about lifting for some time. Mary Cronk says of universal caesarean section recommending medical colleagues:

They haven't thought of the woman who lives on the third floor of a block of flats with two toddlers and a pushchair – they don't think of the impact on the woman of major abdominal surgery. (70)

There are also longer term risks due to scarring of the uterus, including decreased fertility, miscarriage, ectopic pregnancy, placenta abruptio (premature separation of the placenta), placenta accreta (an abnormally adherent placenta which may not detach after birth and may grow through the walls of the uterus) and placenta praevia (the attachment of the placenta to the lower uterine segment) (307). Uterine rupture is a small risk for subsequent labours. Helen contacted me to tell me her experience of an attempted vaginal birth of her second baby (who was head down) after an elective caesarean for her first baby, Caitlin, who was breech:

"I laboured at home for about 21 hours, with the help of my much trusted private midwife, but after all this time was only 3cm dilated. The midwife then advised we should go to hospital, after 11 or so further hours (after pessaries, inducement drips, lots of gas and air and an epidural which did not stem the pain at all of contractions that had no beginning or end) my uterus ruptured (which I felt and knew something bad had happened!). I was given a very necessary emergency caesarean. I woke up some hours later to the sight of another very beautiful baby girl in the cot next to me. Funnily enough, even though the experience sounds and was, at some points, very distressing (much more so for my husband that for me I might add) I came out of that birth viewing the experience much more positively. But feeling much more that it was the first birth experience and lack of information that caused my second delivery to end in the rupture and therefore the second caesarean."

There are also risks to the baby from caesarean section. There is a 6% chance for non-head down babies, as opposed to a 1.9% chance for a head down baby that the surgeons knife will accidentally cut the baby (266). This may go unnoticed: in one study only 1 of the 17 cuts was recorded by the obstetrician (266). There is also the graver risk of respiratory distress for which caesarean section is a "potent risk factor" (307). In a study of 30,000 births, pulmonary hypertension was almost five times higher in babies delivered by caesarean than in babies delivered vaginally (172). A related risk factor is prematurity – even with scanning there are still errors in the timing of elective caesareans which are supposedly done at 38 weeks. Both respiratory distress syndrome and prematurity are major causes of neonatal morbidity and mortality (172). Both of these can be avoided by performing caesarean section after labour has started (see below).

WHY YOU MIGHT WANT A CAESAREAN BIRTH

There are some women who are unmoved or even relieved at the prospect of a caesarean section. If you are very clear that caesarean seems to be a safer option for breech birth the decision to have one may feel very straightforward. Claire contacted me with the following account of her decision making process:

"I asked what would be the safest method [of delivery] for my baby, and I was told that a caesarean would be. I was fully informed of the risks of both options. I am not aware of any reason why I shouldn't have selected the safest path."

Anne's first baby, Rebecca, was breech and born by caesarean section. Her second baby, Edward, was born vaginally after a difficult labour following induction at 38 weeks for reduced amniotic fluid. Although it should be remembered that induction often starts labour off on a difficult footing, more likely to require subsequent intervention, and consequently less likely to be a natural, positive experience for the woman, Anne's opinion is still important:

"I believe that natural childbirth is greatly overrated and NO, I didn't recover more quickly. The only advantage that a 'normal' delivery had over the caesarean was the ability to drive a car. I have a small scar from my caesarean and had no pain post two weeks. With my normal delivery I had pain for weeks after and am very reluctant to have sexual intercourse. I don't think my pelvic floor will ever be the same again."

V. Iovine, American author of *The Best Friend's Guide to Pregnancy*, describes the perceived advantages of caesarean section and why some women opt for it even without a medical need:

With a scheduled caesarean section you and your doctor have agreed a time at which you will enter the hospital in a fairly calm and leisurely fashion, and he or she will extract your baby through a small slit at the top of your pubic hair. There are a lot of reasons to schedule a caesarean section – other women elect to have them because they want to maintain the vaginal tone of a teenager, and their doctors find a medical explanation that will suit the insurance company. (141a)

However, it is important to balance these views with this comment from an American doctor who has written on the subject of women choosing caesarean section:

A woman who chooses CS as a means of avoiding the "biblical sentence to a painful childbirth" is badly misinformed. By choosing a CS she exchanges 12 hours of labour pain for severe post-operative pain and debility and a longer recovery period with weeks or even months of pain. (307)

In relation to the pelvic floor, popularly believed to be protected by caesarean section, evidence appears to suggest no benefit of caesarean over vaginal delivery. In a recent study of Brazilian women, it was pregnancy, rather than the route of delivery, which made women vulnerable to developing urinary incontinence problems (97).

There are many obstetricians who view caesarean as a safer option for breech. Interestingly, Yehudi Gordon, previously a champion of natural active birth for breech, also shares this view: "There is no doubt in my mind that caesarean is safer for the baby provided it's not done too early" (i.e., later than 38 weeks). He believes that vaginal breech birth is always unpredictable, because you can always get cord compression (this issue is discussed in detail in Chapter 10). As a result, he says "that anxiety, that needing to keep your finger on the pulse from minute to minute will never go away" (123). Nigel Saunders, a consultant obstetrician in Southampton and author of a couple of review articles on breech, declined to be interviewed for the book due to time pressure but wrote to me saying: "Ultimately my view is that it is the woman's decision regarding mode of delivery but my personal preference would be for caesarean section" (250). Guy Thorpe-Beeston believes that caesarean section is safer from the baby's point of view and believes that there are more potential complications in a vaginal breech delivery than in a head down one (293). However, he does add that opting for a vaginal breech delivery is still reasonable if the woman satisfies the selection criteria (see Chapter 9).

It may be that you would like to have a natural active breech birth but cannot find a way of negotiating this. If there are no experienced independent midwives in your area, or you cannot afford one, or your local hospital has no-one with appropriate experience and the medicalised option for breech birth feels undesirable and unsafe, caesarean section may start to feel like the only option. Michel Odent expresses his own concerns about the problems of vaginal breech birth with anxious or inexperienced birth attendants: "Breech birth by people who are scared of breech birth can be very dangerous." He continues: "If you are with someone who is scared by breech birth, it is better to let them follow their strategy....It is better to have a caesarean section than to have a difficult birth with someone scared who will do it to please you" (212).

EMERGENCY RATHER THAN ELECTIVE CAESAREANS

It could be argued that there are in fact four types of caesarean section. The first is a true elective section, performed at around 38 weeks. The next is an elective or planned section carried out after labour has started. The third is an unplanned though not urgent "emergency" section, and the fourth is a true emergency section carried out in a considerable hurry after labour has started. Chapter 11 deals with the pros and cons of emergency caesarean in detail. Although you may prefer the certainty of knowing when your baby is coming that an elective caesarean provides, it is worth considering the following arguments.

Babies who have experienced some labour also experience some of the positive "stress" of being born – their hormonal levels (which facilitate breathing) fall somewhere between the optimal levels of babies born vaginally and the less optimal levels of those babies born by elective section. Michel Odent argues strongly for caesarean occurring after labour has started (see Chapter 11). He believes that allowing babies to signal when they are ready to be born is of critical importance and suggests that women due to have a caesarean should state: "I accept the principle of caesarean section but I would like my baby to be ready to be born" (212). Alice Coyle, independent midwife, suggests the use of the term "planned caesarean section at the beginning of labour" for those women who know they want a caesarean but wish to get the benefits of their labour starting (69).

There is also evidence that caesarean scars on wombs already thinned by labour heal more strongly than a scar on a womb that has not laboured at all. This makes the scar less likely to rupture subsequently. It is also believed that when a cervix has effaced and dilated, it will make subsequent labours far quicker and easier. Since many women accept a caesarean for a breech in the hopes that their baby will be head down in a subsequent pregnancy and a normal vaginal birth will be possible, this information is important to decision making.

The main problems with emergency caesarean are that your labour may progress too quickly for a caesarean to be possible (though your labour would need to be unusually rapid for this to be the case), and that the risk to women appears to be higher, though not as high as is sometimes stated. The most recent research estimates the level of risk of infection and other complications as twice that of an elective section for all babies, not only those in a breech position. The difficulty with interpreting this information is understanding the possible reasons for it, again discussed in more detail in Chapter 11. There is a real possibility that the risk of complications is increased by women having urgent emergency sections – those that are done rapidly because the health of the mother or the baby is threatened. Such surgery may be performed with less care and consequently lead to more problems subsequently. If, as is argued in Chapter 11, this is a rare occurrence in breech labours, a study of emergency caesarean section outcomes for breech babies specifically may be better than the general figures would suggest. Thus, if you are planning to have a section after labour has started (which could, perhaps confusingly, be termed an "elective emergency caesarean"!) it may be that this is no less safe than a true elective caesarean. We just don't know.

WHERE YOU WANT TO HAVE YOUR BABY

Which hospital?

You have the right to transfer to a different hospital if you are not happy with the options being presented to you by your current hospital. The next chapter deals with this in more detail.

Private or National Health Service facilities

Some of the women who contacted me had a positive experience of vaginal breech birth after transferring their care to a private hospital. Private hospitals do not take a more open and flexible attitude to being breech just by virtue of being private. Indeed, many private hospitals may have similar or even higher rates of caesarean than NHS hospitals. However, there are places that have attracted clusters of like-minded obstetricians who have developed a culture of natural active birth. The Garden Hospital maternity unit was one of these, but many of the staff from the birth unit there moved to the St John and St Elizabeth in North London (contact details can be found in the Useful Contacts section at the back of this book).

The biggest problem with "going private" is the cost. This is far more expensive than an independent midwife, and it is also important to establish the costs of any unplanned events. A booking for a vaginal birth may seem affordable, but an emergency caesarean may break the bank. Even if a hospital does not charge much more for a caesarean, the normal requirement of a five day hospital stay could increase costs dramatically. It is also worth establishing that the hospital's surgical and intensive care facilities are adequate. Recent attention in the media has focussed on these aspects of private healthcare not always being up to scratch.

I will describe two women's decisions to go private. Both were carrying their first babies and both had been offered a forceps delivery or an elective caesarean section. Jenny takes up the story from there:

I did not consider myself to be evangelical. I had been to ante-natal classes run by the local NCT branch and had read around the subject. I had written a birth plan which indicated that I did not rule out using painkillers but would ask for them if and when I needed them....I talked these developments through with my NCT teacher who suggested I talk to someone who had been through a similar experience. It helped enormously and opened up my options considerably. I realised that I could get a second opinion! My husband and I went to see another obstetrician, Yehudi Gordon[1] for an exploratory chat and advice. He was very reassuring and did not use the scaremongering tactics previously encountered at our local hospital....His unit had a wealth of experience in delivering breech babies without intervention. He encouraged us to take a look around the maternity unit and get to know some of the midwives before making a decision....

Using him would mean 'going private'. It would also mean driving to Hendon (over 20 miles away) for the delivery. I rang BUPA and was told that if my baby was born breech, there would be some cover (room costs, but only a token payment towards the obstetrician's fees). If the baby turned prior to delivery, there would be no cover from my private healthcare plan!

The possibility of changing carers so late in the pregnancy felt a very scary decision to make. My husband and I talked it over and decided that we *should* make the change. At 38½ weeks, we switched from NHS to private, from 5 minutes away to around 35 minutes away (assuming no traffic problems on the A1(M) into London)....

The quality of care was much more sympathetic. My delivery was not treated as a crisis looming over a drama. I was able to spend much of my labour in a birth pool, having been advised to get onto dry land for the actual birth (using gravity). I was gently guided to deliver in a standing squat position with my husband playing an active role in supporting me. When Natasha was born (in my private room with en suite facilites), we were allowed to sit holding her until

1. Yehudi Gordon now works at the St John and St Elizabeth Hospital in North London. He now prefers elective caesarean section for breech birth. However, there are other consultants at the same hospital who are supportive of vaginal breech.

the cord stopped pulsating and my husband was invited to cut it. We were left in peace for a few minutes before I was stitched. The light level was low.

BUPA footed some of the bill, but we had to pay around £1200 (in 1991). We considered it money well spent and still do today. It is more to do with irrevocable experience than purely monetary considerations.

Jenny's second baby, Toby, was head down but she and her husband decided to opt to go private again. She concludes: "I was very fortunate with both my children to have had such a superb quality of care. I fear the outcomes would have left far more traumatic memories had we not decided to make the change."

Fran had felt unhappy about her NHS consultant's approach and went to talk to her NCT teacher

who came up with a third option – change hospitals! She told me about Yehudi Gordon, practising privately in Hendon. I made an appointment, went to see him and was saved. As I remember, his words were something along the lines of "it seems to me you just want to have a go", which was precisely right. I would, of course, have a c-section if it was necessary but I had not been convinced that it was, certainly not at 38+ weeks anyway....

The birth was everything I wanted it to be…I was surrounded by supportive carers in all senses and I never hesitated in my belief that I could do it. I gave birth in a supported squatting position which at the time was fine although I did have an episiotomy as Rosie's heart rate was dipping significantly at the end of the second stage. Rosie was fine…as was I. Lying back in the bath sipping champagne looking at my newly born first child in her father's arms has to rate as one of my most joyous moments in life so far…closely followed by births number 2, 3 and 4. And part of that joy was euphoria that I had followed my instincts and been proved spectacularly right (in my eyes anyway) – it was a seminal moment in my path to becoming an independent midwife myself.

With her independent midwife hat on, Fran reflects on the experience thus:

There is clear evidence that the simple act of having constant support in labour makes significant differences in intervention rates (epidurals/instrumental deliveries, etc.) and now as a midwife it is something I am constantly aware of. Supporting a woman's deepest instincts and giving encouragement enables her to have the confidence to go with those feelings…it is an upward spiral that so often results in a fulfilling, safe and positive birth experience.

It strikes me with some sadness as I read these accounts that such apparently optimal birth experiences simply did not appear to be available for these women on the NHS.

Serious changes of location

The choice of birthplace covered in the rest of this section concerns changes from hospital to home or from one hospital to a different one. Jenny, quoted above, expressed some trepidation at the 30 minute increase in her journey time as a result of changing hospitals.

However, some women make major changes to their planned place of birth in their pursuit of optimal conditions for a vaginal delivery. These changes may be within national boundaries, or may involve leaving the country. There is nothing to stop you arranging a transfer to another part of the country to have your baby with a consultant (NHS or private) or independent midwife whom you have faith in (see Chapter 13 for a more detailed discussion of the process of transferring). Jane Evans told me about a woman who wanted to give birth to her breech baby and was unable to find a hospital or midwife willing to help her near to where she lived. Prior to making contact with Jane, she had been planning to camp in another part of the country near to an independent midwife known to be experienced with breech (94).

Internationally there are places which have become known for a particular approach to breech birth which may appeal to you.

The Farm in Tennessee is a self-sufficient community where babies are delivered by midwives in a home style environment in over 90% of cases. A report by Ina May Gaskin in 1994 showed that of 1888 babies (head down and breech) born over 14 years, only 11 babies died from neonatal complications, and of these, 4 had congenital defects incompatible with life (112). This gives them the highest safety record in America. In her book *Spiritual Midwifery*, she reports 60 successful breech births, none of which needed to be referred to hospital for a caesarean section. It would appear from her statistics that none of the breech babies presenting at the Farm experienced negative outcomes (113). They offer a team of midwives experienced in delivering breech births. Although their approach is natural, it is questionable whether it is active in that most of their breech births seems to take place with the woman in a semi-seated position, and it is certainly not "hands off" – the midwife holds the baby and appears to gently wiggle it out (see Chapter 10). The Farm has produced a remarkable video of 6 breech births which serves as a graphic testament to their approach and makes fascinating and moving viewing. The video can be obtained from the Farm (see the Useful Contacts section). The Farm has women arriving from all over America and may be open to enquiries from the UK vis-a-vis a breech birth. The only difficulty is the issue of flying which is normally advised to stop after 6–7 months. However, it may be possible to negotiate with an airline, as contacts tell me that this cut-off is not hard and fast.

The other international site of particular interest is the Henry Serruys Hospital in Belgium which offers water births for breeches. Further information about their approach is included in Chapter 10 under the heading "The use of water in vaginal breech labour and birth". The contact details are at the back of this book in the Useful Contacts section.

Clearly such a dramatic change of location so late on in pregnancy when for many women energy levels may be dipping and a "nesting instinct" is supposed to be kicking in is a major upheaval. For many women, family commitments or financial issues may make this impossible. However, it has been done. Michel Odent's book *Birth Reborn* includes a woman's account of her decision to transfer from England to his hospital at Pithiviers in France (213). Although Odent has now left Pithiviers and its reputation for natural active birth has ebbed away, the woman's account of her decision making process is interesting and worth recounting in detail:

After two normal births during which I had, nonetheless, suffered all the standard interventions of conventional obstetrics, I was determined that my third delivery would be different. If all went well, I was prepared to find a midwife and insist on a home birth. But an ultrasound scan confirmed that the baby was breech at thirty four weeks, and no-one was confident that it would turn. The doctor at the local hospital suggested that a date be decided upon for me to be induced and said that an epidural and forceps would be used. If that didn't work, I understood that caesareans were quite common for breech babies.

The old depression returned. I had desperately wanted this baby's birth to be natural, and there was no choice of hospital other than the same one that had all the associations of the last confinement, when I felt that the baby had been taken from me....now my hopes for a better experience seemed doomed. This was to be, to my mind another "factory baby".

I had heard about Pithiviers; I knew that women traveled there from other countries. However, I could hardly envisage it as a real possibility for me – I was now 37 weeks pregnant. Still, I rang Dr. Odent a few days later when I had decided that I would regret it forever if I did not gather my strength and make an effort to go to Pithiviers. I asked if I could come. He said, "Why not?" When I said that the baby was breech, he replied "It makes no difference". I immediately felt confident and energetic about the proposed journey.

My husband and I knew very well that time would be short if an emergency arose. Set against this risk was the inevitable recurrence of my depression; before we made the decision to go to Pithiviers, it had already started again. I knew that I could not relive the depression that I experienced after my last confinement and expect to function as a wife and as a mother to three young children....

I suddenly realised that I really had rejected "the system" for the first time in my life. I no longer cared who thought I was making a fuss. I had previously been so polite and helpful to all the medical personnel, and it had got me nowhere – even my own children had been born for me, and this was probably my last chance to take what life has to offer. I just had to take responsibility for myself for a change, and Pithiviers offered an alternative that attracted me. Even its distance appealed to me. I felt a certain animal longing to get away from it all, to have privacy from the people I knew and to find a special place to give birth. I *had* to get to Pithiviers before labour began. This baby was going to be mine and safely mine. I said to my doctor "Things are changing, though, aren't they?" "Yes" he replied, "but that is in a foreign country". My husband informed him later that that was exactly where we were going. (213)

Emotionally, physically and practically it must have taken a lot for this woman to transfer to Pithiviers so late in her pregnancy. What seems to have propelled her most strongly to do it was a sense of how much it would have cost her emotionally if she hadn't.

Breech birth at home

This is not an option that is likely to be discussed with you by your medical team, or indeed by your local midwives. The accepted medical wisdom seems to be that the only breeches that get born at home are undiagnosed ones, and that this is an extremely undesirable state of affairs. Guy Thorpe-Beeston stated: "Anyone can deliver at home if that's their wish, but we can't recommend delivering at home for a breech" (293). Interestingly I heard from two women who were planning home births both of whom had their head down babies misdiagnosed as breech. Both felt that this was related to an "edginess" on the part of the midwives responsible for their care, and both suggested that it would not have happened had they been booked in for a hospital birth.

There are various reasons why some would see giving birth to a breech baby at home as not ideal. It is almost universally agreed that attendance by someone skilled and experienced in breech birth is key to the safety of vaginal breech birth. Experience in breech birth is hard enough to come by in a hospital setting, particularly if the experience you want is of a "hands off" approach to breech birth. However, the fact that breech birth generally takes place in hospitals means that you are more likely to find someone who has at least attended some breech births among the obstetric staff. Unless you are willing to consider an independent midwife, which is discussed in detail in the next section, the chances are that an NHS community midwife is unlikely to have much experience of breech. Wendy Savage commented: "Not only have we got a generation of obstetricians who've hardly seen any vaginal breeches, we've got even more midwives who may never see a vaginal breech" (252). The reasons for having an experienced birth attendant are detailed at the beginning of Chapter 10 and relate in large part to the ability to judge when and when not to intervene. Inexperience can lead to incompetent handling of the birth but can also generate anxiety which may be highly damaging to the woman's confidence in her ability to give birth. It is also important that the birth attendant has the expertise to deliver a breech baby with a nuchal arm (where the arm is caught behind the baby's neck).

The most experienced person you may be able to find in active breech birth may in fact be an independent midwife, so the place of birth does not necessarily determine the level of expertise you can access. Even if you are able to find an obstetrician experienced in breech birth, years of experience with routine epidural and forceps may not be the kind of experience you are looking for.

Many of the arguments people advance for breeches being born in hospital relate to specific facilities that a hospital has that home does not. Donald Gibb argued that cord compression is best monitored using an electronic fetal monitor, only available in hospital (115). This would be disputed by some who would state that intermittent listening with non-electronic means suffices. Michel Odent draws attention to the higher need for emergency caesarean in breech and highlights the convenience factor of an operating theatre being in the same building (212). It is important to remember, however, that the most common reason for section in breech is failure to progress, and that this is generally a decision made with ample time to get to hospital if necessary. Donald Gibb, Caroline Flint and Jane Evans all highlighted the importance of resuscitation in breech births. Many people have pointed out that breech babies may be slower to breathe, more likely to require resuscitation and have lower Apgar scores. Although independent midwives do carry resuscitation equipment, babies may require the help of a neonatologist or paediatrician. Caroline Flint expresses this concern in her own inimitable way: "If you're sitting there with a baby that's very shocked, the most lovely sight in the world is a lovely paediatrician with a lovely resuscitaire!"[2] (103). Jane Evans suggests that breech babies may need resuscitation more often than head down babies because the process of breech birth does not squeeze the fluid from their lungs as effectively as a head down birth. She draws attention to the presence of midwives on labour wards who now specialise in resuscitation and the advantage of accessing their greater skill and experience (94). However, Mary Cronk tells of her frustration when a woman under her care who gave birth in hospital was denied the presence of the resuscitaire in the room because it was hospital policy to keep it at the end of the corridor, in spite of Mary's requests that it be present for the birth. Although the baby was fine, the delay in getting the baby to the machine, and the separation of the woman from the baby immediately after birth were unnecessary (70).

Another concern expressed by both Yehudi Gordon and Donald Gibb, which parallels concerns about becoming overly invested in a vaginal birth, is the danger of allowing an agenda about a home birth take precedence over safety (123, 115). Just as making the emotional adjustment from vaginal birth to emergency caesarean is significant, so too is having to admit that a labour at home would be better off transferred to hospital. However, so long as both woman and birth attendant are prepared for this there is no reason why this should compromise safety. Mary Cronk states clearly that you should not hesitate to transfer to hospital with a breech if all is not progressing well. Although she states there is no evidence to suggest that breech birth at home will lead to poorer outcomes, she cautions against home birth in an isolated setting for this reason (70).

Wendy Savage also points out the higher rates of cerebral palsy in breech babies, regardless of mode of delivery. She says it is important that the woman understands that and isn't going to immediately turn round and find someone to blame if such a tragic outcome occurred in a home birth (252). Caroline Flint, who has had first hand experience of such a traumatic situation in a home birth, comments: "If something happens to the baby, even if it was nothing to do with the birth, the woman will never forgive herself. I don't know if it's worth the risk" (103).

However, some professionals would defend the option of home birth for breech. Alice Coyle, independent midwife, advanced the following arguments for home birth.

The difficulty with hospital is that women are considered to be at risk. In the same way that women having a vaginal birth after caesarean are considered a "trial of scar", women having a breech baby in hospital are considered a "trial

---

2. A resuscitaire is a piece of apparatus with oxygen, suction, a heater, a clock and a flat surface on which to place the baby for resuscitation.

of pelvis". When women are put on trials it is with an expectation of failure. The woman is subjected to much more monitoring than at home, she is confined to the bed more, she doesn't have the freedom to move around or go up and down the stairs and do things which will help the baby and the pelvis. A woman needs to be relaxed and confident to keep her contractions going.With greater access to caesarean section and scanning I don't see why breech at home is so risky. It's the other things about being in hospital that could be risky, especially in a woman who doesn't want to be there. She can have a terribly straightforward labour with a breech just as for a head down baby. You want to give every opportunity for the labour to proceed well – if a woman is feeling safe and protected at home she's far more likely to labour well – if she doesn't you've got plenty of time because the labour tends to just stop. (69)

Jane Evans, independent midwife, makes a similar point about the lack of options for women with breech babies.

At the moment the only place a woman can *give birth* to a breech baby is at home. She can have a vaginal breech extraction in hospital but except in exceptional circumstances the choice is to go in and have interference or to stay at home and give birth to your baby. It's appalling, because you should be able to give birth wherever you feel safest. (94)

There is powerful evidence from detailed statistical analysis carried out by Marjorie Tew, suggesting that home birth may be a safer option than hospital birth, even in high risk cases. Marjorie Tew's book *Safer Childbirth?* provides a devastating critique of the development of the obstetric profession and the corresponding move to give birth in hospital (286). She observed that in the early 1930s, unlike many other conditions in which social class correlated positively with health (the poorer you were the less likely you were to be healthy), maternal mortality appeared to be adversely affected by obstetric care.

Their increased risk of dying from puerperal sepsis as a result of their poorer and less hygienic living conditions was apparently more than offset by their reduced risk as a result of their fewer contacts with doctors....women in the highest social classes were apparently deprived of all their natural advantages of better health and better environment by what was thought to be the best of medical care. (286, p282)

When she studied the move to give birth in hospital and changes in perinatal mortality, she found that the largest declines in infant mortality occurred in areas where the rush to hospital was slower.

Statistics also show that planned home births are the safest of all. Marjorie Tew set out to show whether this could be accounted for by the higher proportion of high risk births in hospital. She excluded from hospital figures any cases which could be considered to be in hospital by virtue of their high risk status so was left comparing like with like: normal booked hospital births with normal planned home births. She found that the hospital mortality rate for babies was 17.3 per 1000, almost three times higher than the figure of 6.0 per 1000 found outside hospital.

The most relevant part of Marjorie Tew's research for women carrying a breech baby is her review of women at all risk levels. It is often assumed that home birth is fine for normal pregnancies but that any risk factor, such as breech makes this unacceptable. The results of her research are presented in Table 12.1.

Table 12.1 Risk prediction and outcome according to place of birth

Labour prediction score	*Mortality rate for babies per 1000 births*	
	GP/midwife	*Hospital*
Very low risk	3.6	8.0
Low risk	4.8	17.9
Moderate risk	2.0	32.2
High risk	14.2	53.2
Very high risk	111.1	149.1
All risks	4.9	27.8

Source: Tew, M. (1998) *Safer Childbirth? A Critical History of Maternity Care*. London, Free Association Books. Reprinted with permission.

Marjorie Tew comments that although in some cases obstetric intervention is lifesaving, these are greatly outweighed by cases where it is not and in fact brings only increased risk. She concludes:

If the objective is to reduce perinatal mortality as quickly as possible, all the evidence already accumulated indicates most cogently that the most immediate and effective method would be to reverse the policy which seeks to ensure that all births take place in obstetric hospitals. (286)

Similar results were found in another review carried out by the National Perinatal Epidemiology Unit in Oxford. They concluded:

There is no evidence to support the claim that the shift to hospital delivery is responsible for the decline in perinatal mortality in England and Wales nor the claim that the safest policy is for all women to be delivered in hospital. (39)

The arguments advanced in Chapter 10 suggest that breech is a prime example of many obstetric interventions being of dubious value (such as forceps, epidural and lithotomy). Some would argue that escaping such interventions by giving birth at home should confer as much if not more benefit in breech birth as head down birth. However, it is important to weigh up this statistical information with the arguments put forward earlier in this section about what hospital may be able to bring to breech birth.

How do women make the difficult decision to give birth to a breech baby at home? There seem to be two broad lines of argument for going for a home birth, which have considerable overlap. The first comes from women who always intended to have a home birth and do not see breech as a valid reason not to go ahead with this plan. Some women who feel this way may have had a previous breech birth and may have great confidence in their ability to give birth naturally. The other line of argument comes from women who do not feel that their hospital can provide the appropriate conditions for a natural active vaginal breech birth. These women will sometimes report feeling forced into giving birth at home, stating a preference for being in hospital with more immediate access to emergency caesarean and neonatal care facilities, but opposing the medical protocol that so often surrounds breech birth in hospital. The reality is that if you feel that you do not want a routine epidural, episiotomy and forceps, and you do want to give birth in an active birth position, you may struggle to find a consultant willing to agree to take you on.

To give you a sense of how some women make the decision to have a breech baby at home it may be helpful to read the following women's accounts of their own decision making. Rachael had her first baby, Florence, at home:

> I had been very single-minded about the birth and stuck out for a home delivery even though I knew the baby was breech and had been criticised for my "irresponsibility" by the hospital obstetrician. I had also had to hold out against the worries of my friends and family who feared for the baby's safety and deal with my own nagging twinges of guilt that I was, perhaps, putting my own needs before the welfare of my child. However, the independent midwives I had hired reassured me that what I felt safest with was most likely safest for the baby. I had felt horrified by the two options offered me by the hospital:
>
> (a) an elective caesarean at 39 weeks
> (b) a trial of labour with "assistance" (i.e., a large episiotomy and forceps).
>
> I also knew that the midwives had good experience of breech deliveries at home and we had looked at photographs and discussed breech labour at great length. So I felt I had taken in the maximum information and prepared my body and mind to the greatest extent I could, and I owed this effort to the child and myself, in order that we should have the best possible chance of an untraumatic labour.

Summing up the context in which Rachael made her decision, she makes an interesting analogy: "There was a mood of doing something illegal – like worshipping in communist Russia! Essential for spiritual well-being but banned by the state!"

Rachael's determination was vindicated by Florence's birth:

> John and I both feel that our own preparations and the expertise and support of our midwives made Florence's birth an empowering and really positive experience for us both. And the best possible way for the baby to come into the world, helped by sensitive and loving experts into the warmth and safety of her own home.

This experience made her decision about her second breech baby far easier:

When I found my second baby was in a breech position at 38 weeks I was unfazed as I had taken the precaution of booking my previous midwives who had delivered my first child. It was expensive but I could not face going through the trauma and anxiety of having to muster adequate care for a breech delivery at the last minute again. Besides the hospital policy would still have been – "on your back, episiotomy and forceps" despite my track record of a short and spontaneous first breech delivery. It was wonderful having the peace of mind that although no. 2 was breech I would be in the best possible hands for a safe delivery at home.

Once again the experience was a positive one with her second child being born 50 minutes after Rachael's waters broke.

Fran had had her first baby, Rosie, in a private hospital (to where she had transferred after feeling hemmed in by the options given to her by her NHS consultant). The birth was a wonderful experience – "everything I wanted it to be" – and second time around Fran booked with an independent midwife with a view to having a home birth. She recounts:

It became increasingly apparent as the pregnancy progressed that Lily too was going to present by the breech. This time I did very little to get her to turn. I felt very relaxed about the whole thing. I had a long discussion with the independent midwives about the increased risks of breech, especially at home. I felt very clear that that was what I wanted to do and refused to go and see the local consultant as I knew he would do lots of shroud waving which I didn't need to hear.

I also felt very clear about the responsibility of my decision. Of course this has not been tested by events but I did do a great deal of thinking about the what ifs, or rather Paul and I did, and came to the conclusion that if there was a problem we would deal with it very much in that context. It's very important to have experienced midwives but that is not the whole story – sometimes nature decides otherwise and my belief is that when you make an "informed decision" consciously then you have to abide by that, whatever the outcome.

Fran's second birth experience was also a joyful one, and very typical of a home birth:

Lily's birth was glorious. My waters went early in the morning, contractions started an hour or so later and I pottered about all morning. I remember lots of laughter and people popping in and out...I progressed well and gave birth standing but leaning into Paul and away from Cath (midwife). I have a great set of photos showing the emergence of Lily which look to me like the laying of the golden egg...initially anyway....Being at home was the icing on the cake and Rosie, who was at the park with her grandmother during the actual birth, was completely unfazed.

Photographs of Lily's birth are shown in the Appendix.

Anne Catt published the story of the birth of her second child, Sadie, who was born breech at home:

My first baby, Jo Louis, was born in hospital, seven weeks premature. Although I wouldn't have been anywhere else under the circumstances, it was a disappointment as I had planned a home birth. I was doubly keen to have the next baby at home, as I find hospitals unnerving – which means that I get all tense and tearful, not conducive to a relaxed, joyful occasion – and staying at home would mean minimum disruption for Jo Louis. (46)

Anne was told to book to see her consultant when Sadie was found to be still lying in the breech position at 37 weeks. However, she stated:

I still wanted to have this baby at home, and felt it would be fine so long as I could find someone confident to be with me. That same day, I got on the telephone to find an independent midwife. The next day, Mary came to see us. Mary is a gale of fresh air. "Of course you can have this baby at home. Breech is not an abnormal presentation, just unusual." We booked her there and then and cancelled the consultant's appointment. As I had not previously delivered a term baby, this was another reason that I had been given for having a hospital birth. "You could get a coach and horses through your pelvis, don't worry about that" [said Mary]. Music to my ears. (46)

Sadie's birth was also a positive experience and in summing it up, Anne draws attention to the central role of the independent midwife in her birth experience: "We would not have booked an independent midwife if Sadie had not been breech. But I am so glad we did. Her birth was everything we could have hoped for."

It is to the issue of who attends the birth of your baby that we shall turn to next.

WHO YOU WANT TO DELIVER YOUR BABY

Midwife or obstetrician

Although many obstetricians would tell you that breech birth should be their domain exclusively, there are those who would disagree. The key seems to be the issue of experience, and Yehudi Gordon is very clear that medical training is not an essential prerequisite to possessing the necessary skills for vaginal breech birth – a process which he suggests is essentially mechanical: "I'd rather have a very skilled midwife doing it than a junior obstetrician" (123). Some would argue that midwives are in fact better placed to help at a breech birth than obstetricians, as does Caroline Flint with her characteristic humour:

obstetricians' mindset is always so much more pessimistic. The baby might die, the mother might die, I might die, we all might die and all that lot! Midwives are much better at just sitting quietly and being quiet. (103)

Alice Coyle agrees that there are certain disadvantages that an obstetrician may bring to a breech birth.

Obstetricians are specialists in the abnormal; they tend to not spend much time with the woman but just come in at the end to do things…We need to get people who are used to dealing with normal vaginal birth to work with vaginal breech instead of people who are used to dealing with instrumental births dealing with vaginal breech which has been a disaster. (69)

Mary Cronk implies that obstetricians should stick with what they are good at: "I'm very grateful for the skills of my medical colleagues in their ability to perform very nice caesarean sections" (70).

There is considerable variation between different consultant obstetricians, however, and the next chapter addresses the issues around trying to find a consultant that you feel happy with if this is the route you choose to take.

An NHS midwife would be prevented by hospital protocol from being the sole birth attendant at a hospital birth. They may attend a breech birth at home though this is often the subject of intense debate between a woman and her local services. As mentioned earlier, it is unlikely that they would have the experience to take on such a role anyway. The complexities surrounding the attendance of independent midwives in hospital are explored below.

Independent midwives

Independent midwives are fully qualified midwives who have chosen to work outside the NHS. They are subject to yearly supervisory visits and equipment checks, and are regulated by the UKCC which require them to keep their practice up to date and act only within their sphere of confidence. You employ one midwife, who would have a back-up midwife if she was unable to attend the birth for any reason. In some situations two midwives may attend a birth together. Independent midwives are normally taken on for a whole pregnancy, but it is not unusual for women to take the route of independent midwifery late on in pregnancy after being disappointed with their standard obstetric care, assuming someone can be found at this late stage (see below). Not all independent midwives would feel comfortable, confident or competent to take on a breech birth at home so it is important that you establish their views and experience of breech from the beginning.

The financial commitment involved in taking on an independent midwife is significant. Mary Cronk expresses women's predicament thus:

Not many of us are in the fortunate position of being able to stump up £2500 [in 2001] without budgeting for it. I would normally say to the woman "You're paying me vast sums of money which you can't necessarily afford and you may end up with a caesarean section." (70)

She also points out that women have at times suffered from extremely hostile reactions from local services in response to contracting with an independent midwife for a home birth for breech. In extreme cases she describes the attitude of some services as being "I wonder if we can get the social workers in – the mother is obviously irresponsible" (70).

The difficulty for independent midwives taking on breech births comes from two sources. The first is from women themselves acting in the current climate of litigation. Caroline Flint states: "Although most breech babies come out perfectly healthy and happy, if the baby comes out dead or damaged, the parents will sue" (103). Although parents may often be driven by noble motives, such as funding the lifetime needs of a child with cerebral palsy, the net effect of the increases in litigation is to make some midwives reluctant to take on breech births. One independent midwife I spoke to has twice been through litigation related to breech birth. Although on neither occasion was her management of the labour and birth itself found to be fundamentally flawed, she has stopped taking on breeches (and the occasional one that slips through the net she insists on taking to hospital). Insurance companies are now imposing high premiums on independent midwives, or are refusing to insure, making their practice more and more difficult.

The second source of difficulty comes from within the midwifery profession. Midwifery bodies are not always supportive of midwives who choose to take on cases that are outside the norm, and there have been cases where attempts have been made to strike off midwives who make these choices.

In addition to these issues which make the climate a somewhat hostile one for independent midwives taking on breech births, one independent midwife I spoke to expressed a reluctance to take on a woman who approaches her late in pregnancy with a breech:

The difficulty is that when women come to us for a "fix-it", they're hoping the baby will turn and will then go back to the NHS to save money. It's not clear when she'll make a decision to stay with us. I don't like to work that way.

Another pointed out the difficulty of taking on a woman at the last minute when "so much of ante-natal care involves getting to know a woman and working out what makes her tick, finding out what's important to her and what isn't". However, most of the independent midwives I spoke to said that they would not turn a woman away in such circumstances. One midwife told me that although she would never lower her fees for late bookers, that if breech was the path that the woman had taken to learning about independent midwifery, that was perfectly acceptable to her.

Independent midwives in hospital

At first glance the option of taking an independent midwife into hospital might appear to be an ideal one. You guarantee the presence of an experienced birth attendant while not denying yourself access to the facilities that a hospital can offer, should these be necessary. The difficulty is that hospitals vary greatly in the respect they accord to independent midwives, with some being welcoming and others refusing to provide an honorary contract. The independent midwife needs an honorary contract in order to practise in the hospital. Without one she can accompany you to the hospital but once there you are likely to be attended by hospital staff as normal. Even hospitals that are normally welcoming of independent midwives may refuse to provide a contract for a breech birth, saying that breech births have to be managed by medical protocol.

Alice Coyle points out that a supportive director of midwives is crucial in this situation "to sort out the doctors" (69). Even if you have found a supportive consultant, this may be of no value if they are not on call when you go in.

Breech births with an independent midwife in hospital are possible though, and can be a positive experience. Rachael had her fourth breech baby (her third had been her only head down baby) in hospital with an independent midwife. Because of the midwife's bad experiences of breech birth at home, the midwife insisted on the birth taking place in hospital. Rachael described the experience thus:

I felt sad to go to hospital but because I recognised how privileged I had been to have had a midwife putting her reputation at risk for me by allowing my first and second births to take place at home, I felt I owed it to her to go. We got a lovely big room – had the baby in two hours without interference or need of a paediatrician, and were home again in bed soon after.

Rachael, though, was not immune to the potential for interference that being in hospital brought.

Although I birthed quickly and successfully with the fourth I wasn't pushing in a creative and primitive manner alone (like with number two), I was pushing in a savage "I can bloody do this, it hurts a lot but it's my way of doing it so – leave us alone!"

There is a definite sense of Rachael having lost something by the transfer into hospital:

One thing I know is that my best breech birth, the second, was made so because it had an ordinary atmosphere surrounding it – no panic, no unfamiliarity. It was sad for me that with the fourth an element of how "wrong" this was crept back in.

SUMMARY

This chapter addresses the issues around the various decisions planning a breech birth raises. Reasons women may want to aim for a vaginal birth include a more rapid recovery time for the mother, avoiding major abdominal surgery, the strength of the mother's own instinct and need to give birth to her child vaginally, and benefits for the baby from experiencing labour which facilitate breathing in the first few hours of life. Reasons for aiming for a natural active birth include the use of gravity and the greater pelvic dimensions created by an active birth position.

Reasons for caesarean include a possible increase in safety for the baby (though depending on your reading of the evidence presented in Chapter 8 this can be seen as unproven) and the mother's own preferences. Even if you are clear that you wish to have a caesarean, you may wish to consider the option of delaying this until labour has started and having a section part way through labour rather than an elective operation. Some have argued that this confers significant health benefits to your baby and promotes stronger scar healing. However, this needs to be weighed against the possible higher risks of complications for you and the possibility that your labour may progress too quickly for a caesarean to be possible.

The place of birth may not be an issue but if you are not happy with what is being offered to you at your local hospital you may want to consider your other options. These include transferring to another hospital, either private or NHS, considering transferring to another centre overseas, or considering giving birth at home. The likelihood is that if you investigate the latter option you will need to consider employing an independent midwife who is experienced in breech delivery. Independent midwives can come with you into hospital but the amount of autonomy they are given varies. Although breech birth is traditionally the domain of obstetricians, it has been suggested that midwives may be as good or better at dealing with breech birth. The most important factor seems to be experience.

Guy Thorpe-Beeston, obstetrician, emphasises that it is ultimately a personal choice for the woman and her partner: "So long as you make clear all the options with the pluses and minuses people will come to a reasoned decision about what to do" (293).

13
Negotiating for the Birth you Want

INTRODUCTION

As with the last chapter, if your decision is to go along with what your consultant advises, there may be little negotiating to do. However, even with a caesarean there are issues about timing and the circumstances in which it is done. You may want to write a birth plan and some suggestions for this are given towards the end of this chapter. If your negotiating task is more major, I hope this chapter provides you with a clear idea of your rights and some hints about how to go about trying to get the birth situation you want. It is important to bear in mind the very real possibility that when negotiating for a vaginal breech birth you may end up with a caesarean section because the labour does not progress well, no matter how ideal the circumstances you have created. Disappointing though this is, many women feel that, if they have been given the optimal conditions for a trial of labour, adjusting to a caesarean is made easier by their knowledge that it was an entirely necessary intervention.

DELAYING AN ELECTIVE CAESAREAN SECTION

There are many reasons why you may want to delay an elective caesarean, either until your due date or until after your labour has started. You may want your baby to be as mature as possible before being born and may want some of the advantages for your baby and for you of experiencing labour. However, you will need to weigh this up against the risks to you of an emergency caesarean section. These issues are discussed in more detail in Chapter 11.

It would not be unfair to say that hospitals and doctors have an inevitable bias towards elective rather than emergency caesarean section that is based on more than just safety. An elective caesarean section at 38 weeks can be performed at a scheduled time and does not involve being called in the middle of the night or at the weekend. It is dramatically more convenient and predictable for all concerned. You may be faced with arguments that an emergency caesarean will harm you more than an elective and that it would be far more sensible to go with an elective operation at 38 weeks. Do make sure that you have read the pros and cons presented in Chapter 11 as it is important that you make up your own mind on this issue. As with so many other breech issues, it is unlikely that you can guarantee having an impartial discussion about it with your medical team.

NEGOTIATING FOR A VAGINAL
BREECH BIRTH/DELIVERY IN HOSPITAL

It is at this stage where the difference between a medically managed vaginal breech delivery and a spontaneous active breech birth becomes key. Simply finding a consultant who is willing to support your baby being born vaginally may not be enough – it is important that you clarify exactly how the birth will be approached.

It is unlikely that you will be able to persuade a consultant who believes that caesarean is the best option for breech and always follows this policy that on this occasion what he really wants to do is a vaginal delivery. Indeed, even if you could it is questionable how desirable this would be. Michel Odent says:

> If you are with someone who is scared by breech birth it is better to let them follow their strategy…it is better to have a caesarean section than to have a difficult birth with someone scared who will do it to please you. (212)

This then leaves you facing the option of changing consultant or hospital which is dealt with in the section below.

However, the key to negotiating for a vaginal birth carried out in the way that you choose is clear communication. In order to transfer hospitals or consultants you need to be very clear that your current consultant is not willing to support you. Although it may be obvious in some cases, in others the issue may be less clear. One woman's experience shows the importance of being clear and persistent:

> I asked my consultant if I would be supported in giving birth in a position of my choosing such as standing, all fours or laterally. He smiled and said benignly "You can assume whatever position you wish my dear." I was impressed by his permissiveness but this was too important an issue to be fudged: one of my biggest fears was being in labour and having to fight my way through the birth. "So just to clarify," I said, "are you saying that the medical team will support me in delivering the baby on all fours, for example?" He replied: "Well for second stage, of course, we will need you to be in lithotomy, so that we can use forceps – it is terribly important to control the birth of a breech."

One way of ensuring that communication is clear is to write a birth plan and go through it with your consultant point by point (see the section below on birth planning). Another is to ask some of the following questions:

- How many planned vaginal breech births have you attended in the last year?
- How many of these ended up in an emergency caesarean?
- Have you attended any vaginal breech births where delivery occurred in a standing/squatting/all fours position? If so, how many?
- What are your views on this way of giving birth to a breech baby?
- Do you routinely use forceps and lithotomy in breech labour?
- Do you routinely use an epidural in breech labour?
- Do you routinely use an episiotomy in breech birth?

- What are your views on electronic fetal monitoring in a breech labour? (If the consultant feels it should be used routinely, or is likely to be necessary, you may want to check how willing he is for you to be in an upright position during monitoring.)
- What are your views on augmentation in a breech labour?

TRANSFERRING HOSPITALS/CONSULTANTS

Wendy Savage illustrated the importance of your consultant's attitude to breech. Even in a hospital which essentially supports vaginal delivery of breech babies, her own rate for vaginal breech birth is 2 in 3 attempted vaginal deliveries, one colleague's is 1 in 2 and another colleague's is 1 in 3. So, she points out, "you can have your chance of a vaginal delivery doubled depending on who your consultant is" (252).

Initially you may not see your consultant. You have a right to see him or her, and if this is not offered to you automatically when your baby is diagnosed as breech, you can ask to make an appointment with them. Donald Gibb cautions that "some of the more junior consultants are just older junior doctors who have no experience of vaginal breech" (115). If you are not happy with your consultant's approach, you can ask: "Is there another consultant in this hospital who might take a different view?"

If you cannot find a consultant in your local hospital who is experienced in and sympathetic to breech birth, you may wish to start looking further afield. Ask around – local midwives or ante-natal class teachers may have a good idea of hospitals in your area that take a more favourable approach to breech. They or your GP should certainly be able to give you the location of other obstetric hospitals in the vicinity. Once you have a list of obstetric hospitals that you wish to get in touch with, the person to contact is the Director of Midwifery Services. They will have a good knowledge of the approaches taken by the different consultants at their hospital and will help you to arrange an initial appointment if you wish to. There is nothing to stop you contacting more than one Director of Midwifery services at any one time. As time is of the essence at this stage and if you have more than one lead, you can do your research in parallel. If anyone makes any objection, remind them that you have a right to a second opinion. If you find someone you feel is right for you and who has agreed to take you on, you ideally should arrange for your consultant, GP or midwife to refer you. Wendy Savage said that she would have been willing to accept someone who has not managed to get a referral, but that life is easier if such a situation can be avoided.

Finding a sympathetic consultant is not the end of the road, however. Although your consultant's view is likely to affect the prevailing culture of your care, you may also want to ensure that you have spoken with the registrar as well. In one study more than 80% of breech births were attended by the registrar rather than the consultant (265). So there is a scenario where you could have a consultant who is supportive of active vaginal breech birth and a registrar who is more conservative. If you have any concerns about this you can raise it directly with your consultant. You can request that he/she is present at your birth and although you do not have a right to insist on it (if you are in labour outside of working hours, your consultant may not be on call), he/she may be happy to be in telephone contact if he/she is not actually present. The same concern arises in relation to the staff on duty when your labour starts. Unless your consultant/registrar are willing to be present or offer telephone support even when they are not on duty, you may be faced with a team managing you with a different approach which undermines all your attempts at negotiation in advance. It is worth asking your team about this. If your consultant and registrar are the only ones supportive of vaginal breech in that hospital, you need to talk through with them what they can do to ensure that it is their management style which governs your labour. As above, it may be that they are willing to be in telephone contact if they will not attend the labour.

Although it may feel a little harsh to be asking your doctor to be on duty when he is not working, there are not many situations in obstetrics that have the same dependence on an individual doctor's attitudes. It seems fairly unacceptable that your care is determined by individual variation to the extent that it is, and in this context, if you have found someone whom you trust with your care, it seems reasonable to try to ensure his/her influence over your birth rather than a colleague whose views may be sharply opposing to their own. You can also rest assured that this is a situation that arises rarely. Breech represents only 3% of births (some of which are undiagnosed until after labour has started). Many women opt for a caesarean section. So it is unlikely that any one consultant will be dealing with more than a handful of requests per year at the most to be available for a vaginal breech.

BREECH BIRTH AT HOME

AIMS (Association for Improvements in Maternity Services) has produced an excellent booklet on choosing a home birth from which much of the information in this section is drawn (288). Their contact details are provided at the back of this book in the Useful Contacts section.

Every woman has the legal right to give birth at home, regardless of any perceived risk factors. It had been thought that your local health authority has a legal obligation to ensure that you are attended by a qualified practitioner (usually a midwife), but at the time of writing this is under discussion, with some trusts attempting to refuse on the grounds of staff shortages. AIMS will have the latest position on this (see Useful Contacts section at the end of the book). The Health Authority is not legally required to provide GP cover for a home birth. The midwife (or team of midwives) must provide full ante-natal, birth and post-natal care. Midwives do not require GP backing in order to provide care. If medical tests or services are needed during pregnancy, the midwife is able to refer a woman booked for home delivery directly to a local hospital for tests.

A midwife called to a woman in labour must attend. Should complications arise in labour the midwife can call on the services of any GP on the obstetric list (i.e., a GP with obstetric qualifications – a rare breed these days), even if they have not been previously involved in your care, or can transfer you to hospital.

You may be asked to sign a disclaimer, relinquishing the hospital or Trust of all responsibility for the outcome. You cannot be forced to sign such a document (your right to give birth at home certainly does not depend on it) and even if you do, these documents are not necessarily legally binding.

If you did not originally plan a home birth but decide late in your pregnancy that you want one, all of the above still applies. Carrying a breech baby does not affect your rights in any way. You do not have to explain or justify why you want to give birth at home if you do not want to.

It is often assumed that your GP should be your first port of call for arranging a home birth. In an ideal world this would be so, and the government report *Changing Childbirth* made it clear that "GPs who feel unable to offer care of support to a woman who wishes to have a home birth should refer the woman directly to a midwife" (237). However in practice it may not be so straightforward. Reports abound of women who have been struck off (or indeed had their entire families struck off) for wanting a home birth, and your GP may work hard to scare you into a hospital birth. You do have the right to find a new GP. One woman went to 12 practices in her attempts to find a supportive GP. You can also remain signed on with your own GP and approach a new GP for maternity care only. Though not all GPs are happy about you doing this (and may strike you off if they are very unhappy) this does not affect your right to do it.

However, to quote Pat Thomas' AIMS leaflet on the subject: "There is no reason – medical, legal or ethical – to involve your GP at all if you want a home birth" (288). You can make a direct approach to your community midwives or to the Supervisor of Midwives/Director of Midwifery, based at the local maternity unit and ask for arrangements to be made for you to be booked in for a home birth. Contact details can be obtained from your local community health council or by telephoning your local obstetric unit.

In a case reported by Beverly Beech in the AIMS journal a woman expecting a breech baby was told by her trust's chief executive that "a home delivery of a breech presentation baby is outside the scope of practice for our midwives and providing sub-optimal obstetric care at home is simply not an option for us". When it was suggested that the Trust should give a temporary contract to an independent midwife who was skilled in breech birth the Trust refused. When the mother said that she was determined to stay at home he announced that in that case the hospital's on call midwives would attend. Mary Cronk suggests the even bolder strategy for women dissatisfied with the level of competence and experience in breech at her local hospital: "The woman should say 'No – I wish to engage a competent prac-titioner and since you can't provide one I shall find an independent midwife and send the bill to the Department of Health'" (70). She did not know of anyone who had succeeded in this, however.

WRITING A BIRTH PLAN

Birth plans are the inevitable result of the failure of "experts" and mothers to communicate with and trust each other. For years medical practice has been justified by insisting that women "never asked for anything different". Women, on the other hand, insisted for years that they have asked, but have not been heard....until things improve, it looks like the birth plan is here to stay. (287)

This is Pat Thomas' view on birth plans, and her conception of it as a response to communication failure in labour helps to focus the mind on the key functions of a birth plan. If your relationship with your care givers is excellent and you know that they will be present at your labour you may feel you do not need a birth plan. However, to avoid having to present your views while in labour it seems like a sensible precaution.

One function of a birth plan, sometimes overlooked, is the way in which it helps you to clarify what matters to you. It is important not to get carried away with your image of your ideal birth: while everything may go according to plan, it may not and it is important to have contingency plans. For example: "I would rather not use medication for pain relief, but if I do feel I need it gas and air would be my preference. If I need something stronger I would prefer an epidural. I do not wish to be given pethidine." Another example of contingency planning is thinking through what may happen should an emergency caesarean become necessary. Ultimately, whatever you write in your birth plan should be viewed as a set of guidelines. If you change your mind about anything in it, you should do so freely and without embarrassment.

It is important not to be "fuzzy" in your birth plan. For example: "I want an active birth" may be open to misinterpretation (deliberate or otherwise). It would be better to state: "I want to move around throughout my labour and wish to give birth in a standing/squatting/all fours position."

Although many women don't get round to writing a birth plan until very late in their pregnancies, it is helpful if you have had a chance to talk through its contents with your birth attendants. If they do have a problem with anything you are suggesting it is far better to know well before your labour starts (when you may have the time to negotiate, or transfer to a different attendant) than after. The advantage of a birth plan is that it forces a greater clarity about people's approach than a general discussion can. For example, a consultant may be in favour of active birth during labour but require a woman to be in the lithotomy position for the birth itself.

Birth plans are not legally binding documents. Your attendants are not obliged to follow your wishes. If you know you are not transferring elsewhere it is worthwhile investing some energy in maintaining friendly relations with your attendants where possible as logic would suggest that this may make them more likely to be willing to go along with your plan. Sheila Kitzinger points out that doctors and midwives can get very anxious about birth plans. She suggests:

You may find you need to reassure them about why you want a birth plan. Explain that you are flexible and will accept intervention if you consider it necessary, and that you are glad to have advice (even though sometimes in the end your conclusion may be different from theirs). (155a)

If you can get your consultant to sign your birth plan this will lend it a credibility which will help if ultimately your labour is managed by someone else.

Caesarean birth plan requests

Here are a list of possible requests you may wish to include in a birth plan. Even if you are not booked in for a caesarean and are hoping to have a vaginal birth it makes sense to include a section on caesarean birth in case you end up having one. Some of the requests below may strike a chord with you, others may not and others you may wish to include in their opposite form (for example, most people feel fairly strongly about whether or not to have a curtain obscuring your view of the operation). This list should be used as a means to clarify your own thoughts, rather than as a model.

I would like to:

- wait for labour to start before the caesarean section is performed
- discuss all procedures in advance
- have my partner with me throughout
- be given medication only after receiving information about it
- have epidural anaesthesia for the operation
- have no curtain obstructing my view
- have a mirror so that I can watch the birth if I wish
- have a commentary on what is happening
- have the theatre as quiet as possible at the moment of birth
- have the lights turned down for a few minutes at the moment of birth
- have the baby delivered straight onto me
- discover the sex of the baby ourselves
- hold the baby immediately after the birth and breastfeed immediately
- if I am under general anaesthetic, have my partner hold the baby immediately
- have the baby stay with me all the time unless he/she needs to be taken elsewhere for medical reasons
- be consulted about it first if the baby needs to go elsewhere
- have a visit from my 3-year-old, and a chance for her to meet the baby, as soon as possible.

Vaginal breech birth plan requests

First stage of labour:

- I would like to start labour spontaneously and not be induced unless it is decided that the baby might be at risk/not be induced at all and have a caesarean if it is decided that the baby might be at risk
- I would prefer oxytocic drugs not to be used unless absolutely necessary/ I would prefer to proceed to an emergency caesarean if my labour is not progressing and not use oxytocic drugs
- My consultant/registrar has agreed to be telephoned when I arrive in hospital if they are not on duty and come in/remain in telephone contact
- I would like to have intermittent monitoring to enable me to move around freely. If labour is prolonged or there are deviations from the norm which

give rise to concern about the baby I am happy to have electronic fetal monitoring for as long as is necessary but would like to remain upright if possible

- If it is felt that the baby is in distress from the evidence provided by the fetal monitoring, I would like this to be confirmed with a blood sample from the fetal buttock
- I would prefer not to have an epidural but recognise that I may need one if I am struggling to cope with the pain. I do not wish to be given an epidural purely to manage my labour. I have practised breathing techniques which should help me manage any premature urge to push. I do not wish to have an epidural or pethidine for pain relief and would want to have an emergency caesarean if I am no longer able to cope with the pain
- I am willing to be catheterised if I am having difficulty urinating and this may be holding up my labour.

Second stage of labour:

- I would like to give birth to my baby in a standing/squatting/all fours position
- I do not wish forceps to be used as a matter of course to deliver the head, unless absolutely necessary
- I would prefer the Mauriceau Smellie Veit manoeuvre [see Chapter 10] to be used to deliver my baby's head
- I do not wish to be given an episiotomy unless it is felt the baby would benefit from it.

Third stage of labour:

- Unless there are serious concerns about my baby's condition, I would like to hold him/her before examination
- I would prefer the cord not to be cut until the placenta has stopped pulsating. My partner would like to cut it. If the baby needs resuscitation I would like the resuscitaire to be placed next to the bed, and to keep the cord intact if possible
- I do not wish to have syntometrine [see Chapter 10] unless it is necessary.

NEGOTIATING IN LABOUR

Clearly most women want to focus solely on giving birth when that is what they are doing, and the thought of negotiating during labour can be horrifying. There is also the real fear that it may not be a time most conducive to assertiveness and that your options are limited: you can hardly opt to go elsewhere midway through labour (though many women have tried!). However, I have heard stories of women who have managed to have the active vaginal birth experience they wanted apparently simply by having a good progressive labour and encouraging their attendants to go with the flow. Beatrice's account of the birth of her daughter, Teri, who was breech, is a good example of this. Beatrice needed to be induced after her waters broke and was given a pessary at noon with the instruction to relax and wait till she was given a second pessary at 6pm. She takes up the story from here.

By 4.30pm I was breaking into a light sweat and counting through the waves of pain. The midwife took a look at me just to be on the safe side…and found I was 10cm dilated and already in the second stage. I knew then that I was home free and felt immediately calm and in control. I insisted on standing and following the heartbeat monitor while laughing and joking between contractions. It was going so well that the senior midwife asked me if her staff could come in and watch. *A couple of doctors joined the fray and there was a terse exchange about my standing position* [my italics], but after a quick flick of the umbilical cord over her head my daughter was born at 6.05pm.

Beatrice seems to have been able to use the power of her progressive labour to almost silence the opposition. Although we don't have details of exactly how her labour had been planned, her tale of overcoming her doctor's objections to standing is a heartening one.

However, using the progress of your labour to help your case for a vaginal delivery, depends both on how your labour develops and on whom you're negotiating with. One woman described a negative experience, in spite of her good progress:

I arrived at the hospital 7½ cm dilated and tried to convince the consultant I wanted to deliver normally…He "talked me round" to having a section. In a way I feel cheated because I wasn't fully in control of myself and I was talked round.

If you are faced with decisions to make in labour, particularly relating to intervention, the following questions may help you with the negotiation process (159).

1. Is this an emergency or do we have time to talk?
2. What would be the benefits of doing this?
3. What would be the risks?
4. If we do this, what other procedures or treatments might we need as a result?
5. What else could we try first instead?
6. What would happen if we waited an hour or two before doing it?
7. What would happen if we didn't do it at all?

The unpredictability of labour means that it is probably best to cover all your bases and do as much negotiating as you can before you are in labour. Then even if you don't get the birth experience you want, at least you can feel that you have done everything in your power to make it possible.

SUMMARY

This chapter tries to address most of the subjects you may need to negotiate on. It briefly discusses delaying an elective caesarean section until after labour has started, and addresses some issues that may arise when you are negotiating for a vaginal birth. The importance of clear communication is emphasised: one person's conception of a vaginal breech birth may be very different to another's. The process involved in transferring to a different hospital/consultant is described, as are your rights to have a home birth. You have a legal right to a home birth and the health authority is legally obliged to provide you with care (usually from a midwife). This is not changed by your baby being breech. The reasons for writing a birth plan are briefly discussed and some suggestions as to what you may wish to include in both a plan for a vaginal and a caesarean birth. Even if you are hoping to have a vaginal birth you may also want to consider writing a plan for a caesarean in case it becomes necessary. The pros and cons of doing your negotiating in labour are also discussed and some examples of women's experiences of this provided.

Epilogue

When I turned up to interview the consultant who had attended the birth of my own breech baby two years before, he had a question for me. Perhaps partly surprised by my continued preoccupation with the subject of breech he asked: "Are you doing this to get it out of you, doing it because you're fascinated and obsessed by it, or doing it because you want people to know about the research and their options?" I replied that it was probably all three combined, plus the perhaps naive hope that the book might make a difference to what was being offered to women out there. He responded: "Regrettably the best reason for doing it is probably no longer relevant – we would like to change people's practices to offer choice but the game may already be over." One of my concerns in writing the book has been that information may be a frustrating possession when local services fail to offer you the options that research and many experienced clinicians suggest should be open to you.

However, there are some encouraging signs that the game may not be over. A survey of registrars' approach to breech in the UK published a few years ago indicated that less than 10% would routinely offer caesarean section for breech and that only 15% would routinely offer section for a first baby (261); a surprising 81% said that they would support vaginal breech birth in a close relative; 40% said that their approach was not dictated by hospital protocol; 60% had been present at more than 20 vaginal breech deliveries. These figures need to be seen in the context of a response rate to the survey of 51%. It is possible that registrars who were more enthusiastic about caesarean delivery for breech did not respond. This survey was also carried out prior to the term breech trial which has been responsible for a dramatic increase in caesarean section for breech, in spite of the study's major flaws. Nevertheless, it suggests that there are registrars out there who are open to vaginal breech birth.

The most accessible area for change is in the arena of turning techniques. Information should be disseminated on alternative techniques for turning breech babies and more research carried out. The Royal College of Obstetricians and Gynaecologists (RCOG) should play a more active role in ensuring that all women have the opportunity to access ECV if they wish to, as the current levels of practice described in Chapter 5 are simply unacceptable.

Accessing active vaginal breech birth is a particular problem as this is still regarded as unacceptable in many hospitals. My first plea for change in this area is for research. Active vaginal breech birth is desperately under-researched and until we have good sized, well designed studies evaluating this approach, vaginal breech birth cannot be declared as riskier than caesarean. The problem is that such research, if carried out properly, requires extensive funding and organisation. I would urge those doctors and midwives who do offer active vaginal breech birth to audit their practice (simply by keeping a record of case details and outcomes) and to publish the results. By becoming more visible to one another, such practitioners may ultimately be able to mount a multi-centre study which may ultimately be able to seriously address the relative safety of active vaginal versus caesarean breech birth.

My second plea is for training. At present it is possible for obstetricians to get through their training without witnessing a vaginal breech birth, and quite likely that midwives will never see one. The chances of seeing a skilled and experienced practitioner attending a spontaneous active vaginal breech birth are even lower. Theoretical training is likely to focus on vaginal breech delivery, often to the exclusion of the principles and techniques involved in active vaginal breech birth. This dying out of breech birth skills is deeply concerning. Two of the people I spoke to for this book (Wendy Savage and Michel Odent) are now retired from clinical work. Women are being forced to opt for caesarean section because their local obstetric services are unable to provide them with a competent birth attendant. The significant proportion of women who experience an undiagnosed breech and/or whose labours are too progressive to resort to caesarean section will generally be attended by panicky and unskilled personnel, who have been known to resort to a caesarean section, even when labour is so advanced to make this an actively risky process for mother and baby (70). Given that undiagnosed breeches will continue to occur, it seems essential for all obstetric and midwifery staff to have appropriate training. This point was picked up in some recent correspondence in the *British Medical Journal* arising from the Term Breech Trial. Varma and Horwell comment:

Obstetricians' inexperience in managing vaginal breech delivery has contributed to adverse outcome and is likely to increase as a result of the current change in practice. Nevertheless, it is impossible to deliver all term breech pregnancies by caesarean section. The mother may insist on vaginal delivery, breech labour may be precipitate, and there are special situations such as the second fetus in twins. It is therefore imperative that trainees continue to receive training in vaginal breech delivery. (301a)

The problem with training is the small numbers of people possessing expertise in vaginal breech birth and its relatively infrequent occurrence. For this reason, I would suggest that at least for an interim period, specialist centres are set up across the country that can centralise resources and knowledge for breech and act as a training resource. Ideally every region should have its own centre, with a view to spreading expertise out to local hospitals and midwifery services. Midwifery outreach teams, able to attend home births, should also be part of such a service development. Regardless of one's view of the wisdom of giving birth to a breech baby at home, women are likely to continue to exercise their right to give birth at home, and it should be the responsibility of services to provide skilled personnel to attend these births.

The RCOG and Royal College of Midwives, in conjunction with organisations such as the Association for Improvements in Maternity Services (AIMS) and the

National Childbirth Trust should play a lead role in the planning and implementation of such training.

Another plea is to allow midwives to become actively involved in the management of vaginal breech birth. The key to attending a vaginal breech birth appears to be experience and specialist knowledge, rather than any particular obstetric skill. As Marsden Wagner comments:

Midwifery uses a different paradigm by focusing not on the potential for abnormality but on the normality of pregnancy. To a midwife a breech birth is a variation of the normal; to a doctor it is a pathological condition. Caesarean section rates are lower when midwives rather than doctors attend the birth. (307)

Jane Evans, independent midwife, is clear that training more midwives in the skills of breech birth is the way forward:

Midwives should stand up and become midwives again. Women need to be up there demanding midwives not obstetric nurses. In countries like New Zealand where midwives have come back it is because women have fought for them and said "No – we're not going to be treated like this anymore, we want to *give birth* to our babies." Midwives get the theory of breech birth but they don't get the practice. They need a practical apprenticeship. (94)

Jean Robinson of AIMS also points out that obstetricians potentially have a lot to learn from experienced midwives like Mary Cronk and has been in conversation with the RCOG to encourage them to consider training opportunities. The outcome of these conversations is eagerly awaited.

In spite of the publication of the Canadian multi-centre breech trial, which some people regard as the basis for recommending universal caesarean section (though should perhaps be regarded more appropriately as a nail in the coffin of medically managed hands (and forceps) on vaginal breech delivery), there are signs that hospitals are nevertheless starting to offer more choice. One consultant told me that up to a few years ago universal section was common practice in Scotland but that things are now changing because people are demanding more options (293). We all have a role to play in ensuring that such demands are made and heard, as women, partners, midwives, ante-natal class teachers and doctors.

It would be easy to give up, to go for a policy of universal caesarean section for breech as the simplest next step. But caesarean section cannot be the response to suboptimal care for vaginal breech birth. More research and training must be the answer, before it is too late.

Useful Contacts

Active Birth Centre
55 Dartmouth Park Road
London NW5 1SL
020 7267 3006

Association for Improvements in Maternity Services (AIMS)
Beverly A. Lawrence Beech
5 Ann's Court
Grove Road
Surbiton KT6 4BE
020 8390 9534
Helpline number 08707 651433

Association of Radical Midwives
62 Greetby Hill
Ormskirk
Lancashire L39 2DT
01695 572776
Website www.midwifery.org.uk
Email arm@midwifery.org.uk

The Association of Reflexologists
27 Old Gloucester Street
London WC1 3XX
The Association publishes a register of qualified reflexologists.

British Acupuncture Council
63 Jeddo Road,
London W12 9HQ
020 8735 0400
Provides a list of qualified acupuncturists, specifying those with a particular interest in pregnancy and birth.

The Farm
The Farm
Summertown
38483 USA
Centre where Ina May Gaskin and her team of midwives practise. Has produced a video of breech births. Willingness to take on women from outside the US would need to be negotiated with staff at the Farm.

Henry Serruys Hospital
Yves De Smedt
Maternity Ward
Kairostraat 84
8400 Oostende
Belgium
058 51 15 58
Hospital specialising in water birth with experience of breech water birth.

St John and St Elizabeth Hospital
60 Grove End Road
London NW8 9NH
020 7286 5126
Private hospital at which Donald Gibb (sympathetic to vaginal breech birth) and
Yehudi Gordon (interested in ECV and alternative turning methods) work – both
interviewed for this book.

Independent Midwives' Association
1 The Great Quarry
Guildford GU1 3XN
01483 821104
Website www.independentmidwives.org.uk
Email info@independentmidwives.org.uk

Midirs
Midwives Information and Resource Service
9 Elmdale Road
Clifton
Bristol BS8 1SL
0117 925 1791
Website www.midirs.org
Email digest@midirs.org.uk

National Childbirth Trust
Alexandra House
Oldham Terrace
Acton
London W3 6NH
0870 4448707
As well as offering nationwide ante-natal classes and post-natal support, the NCT
may be able to put you in touch with women in your area who have had similar
experiences.

WEBSITES

www.BirthChoiceUK.com
A non-commercial website on maternity care options, including details on local maternity services and rights to a home birth.

www.breechbabies.com
A one-woman website designed to bring together information, stories and pictures about breech birth. The woman concerned is a mother, perinatal nurse and birth educator. A fantastic resource.

www.caesarean.org.uk
A non-commercial website devoted to all aspects of caesarean birth and vaginal birth after caesarean (VBAC), including articles, birth stories and photographs of caesarean scars.

www.gentlebirth.org
An American broad-based, helpful but anecdotal website with sections on prenatal breech birth issues (especially turning) and attending a breech birth.

www.midwifery.org.uk
Helpful information on current issues in midwifery and various leaflets for parents and midwives from the Association of Radical Midwives.

Appendix: Birth Photographs

THE BIRTH OF RACHAEL'S BABY, JACK

Jack, Rachael's fourth baby, was born in hospital with an independent midwife. Jack was an extended breech. There is sometimes a false impression given in discussion of active birth positions that a woman chooses her favoured position for birth and sticks to it no matter what. These photographs illustrate the flexibility of positioning and the hybrids of positions it is possible to create.

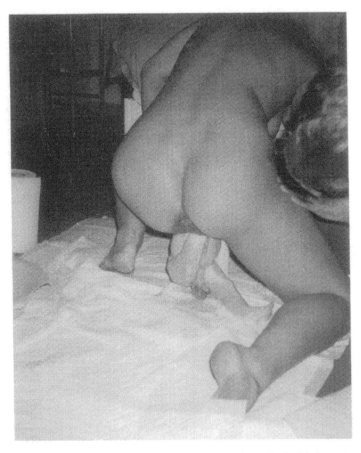

Jack's left leg is fully out, his right is still coming down. Rachael is in a part kneeling, part squatting position. Jack's swollen testicles can also be seen clearly. It is common for testicles to swell during a breech birth. Some people think this protects the testicles from damage during birth.

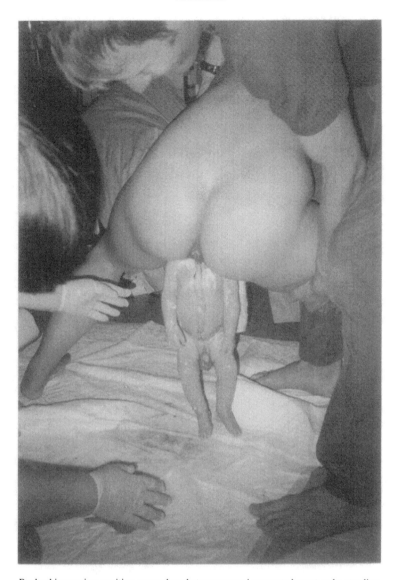

Rachael is now in a position somewhere between a semi-supported squat and a standing position, though her upper body is well forward as it would be if she was on all fours. Jack's body has almost entirely emerged and is hanging. This is the stage, described in Chapter 10 under the heading "Experience of the team", which is thought to require particular experience to manage. The biggest danger for the baby at this stage is likely to be from being pulled out, and its head extending.

THE BIRTH OF FRAN'S BABY, LILY

Lily, Fran's second baby, was born at home with an independent midwife. Lily was an extended breech. Although Fran is standing, it is now common in independent midwifery practice for the woman to be kneeling. Fran's midwife is also handling the baby more than would now be usual.

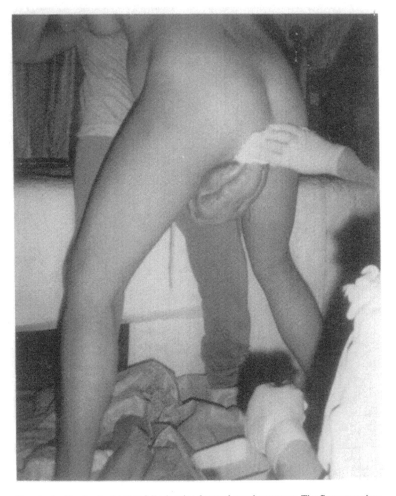

Fran is standing to give birth to Lily, leaning forward onto her partner. The first meconium had already emerged at this point, which is quite normal in a breech birth (see Chapter 10). The baby's bottom has been born and the legs and trunk are now slowly emerging. This photo beautifully illustrates what Mary Cronk describes as "the legs going on for miles"!

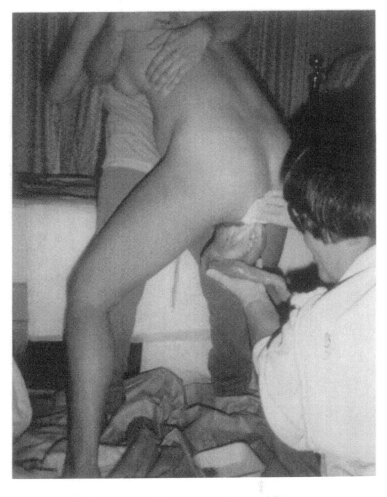

One leg has dropped down. The cord is now visible.

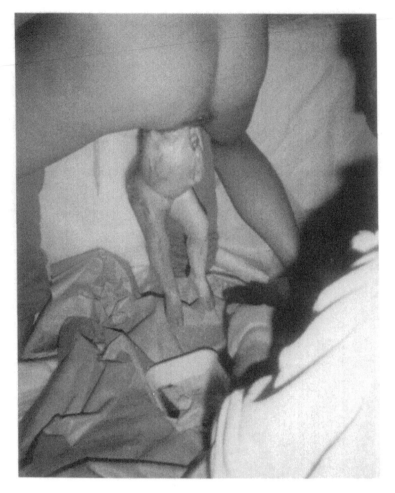

The cord is now clearly visible and both baby and cord have good colour. Both legs are now down but Lily's arms are raised and will need help to be brought down.

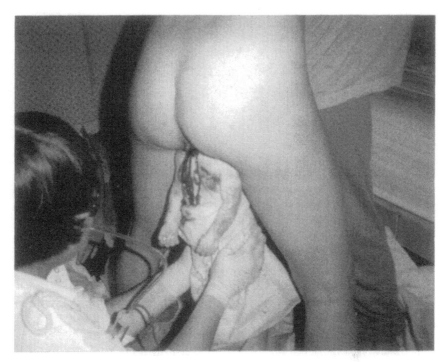

After inserting a thumb to help sweep the arm down, the baby's body has now been fully born. The blood on the baby's chest is quite normal at this stage in any birth. The midwife has her suction apparatus ready, which she will use to insert an airway when the baby's mouth emerges. Although the baby is wrapped, this is not always done and not generally regarded as essential.

Further Reading

BREECH SPECIFIC

AIMS Journal (1998) Special Issue on Breech Birth. Autumn. Volume 10, part 3
This is an excellent resource, including a couple of informative articles by Gina Lowden (already referenced in this book) and some accounts of women's experiences of breech birth, including my own.

Banks, Maggie (1998) *Breech Birth Woman-Wise*. Birthspirit Books, Hamilton, New Zealand. ISBN 0–473–04991–0
Available from Birthspirit Books, 15 Te Awa Road, R.D. 3, Hamilton, New Zealand
Phone New Zealand 64 07 8564612
Fax New Zealand 64 07 8563070
email banks@ihug.co.nz
Unfortunately, Maggie Banks' book has not had the international publicity it deserves, and as a consequence I did not get hold of it until I was well into writing my own book. Written by a midwife, it contains greater detail on the process of vaginal breech birth with lots of photos and diagrams, and has much to offer medical and midwifery students, practising midwives and obstetricians. Coming from a midwife who is deeply woman centred in her approach it also makes highly empowering reading for women and their partners.

Midirs and the NHS Centre for Reviews and Dissemination (1997) *Breech Baby – Options for Care*. Midirs (see Useful Contacts section for contact details)
Both this leaflet designed for professionals and its counterpart designed for women were useful and empowering for me when I was pregnant. The fact that they have been written by a body of professionals and so represent current professional opinion felt particularly reassuring when the professionals immediately surrounding me were presenting different views.

GENERAL

Lagercrantz, Hugo and Slotkin, Theodore, A. (1986) The "Stress" of Being Born. *Scientific American* 254(4): 92–107
I get fed up at the frequent protrayal of normal vaginal birth as an awful trauma for the baby. A recent television documentary made the rather ludicrous comparison to the experience of careering down a ski slope at high speeds (the implication being that it is really far kinder on our babies to opt for a caesarean). This paper provides a welcome antidote to this view, giving a scientifically

supported account of the way in which vaginal birth may help the newborn baby's survival outside the womb.

Sutton, J. and Scott, P. (1996) *Understanding and Teaching Optimal Foetal Positioning*. New Zealand, Birth Concepts
This book is of use to any woman planning a vaginal birth, be it breech or head down to encourage the baby to assume an optimal position. The baby's position as labour starts can make all the difference to your progress.

Tew, Marjorie (1998) *Safer Childbirth? A Critical History of Maternity Care*. Free Association Books, London. ISBN 1–85343–426–4
If you were in any doubt about the extent to which the obstetric profession is evidence based, this book undermines obstetrics from its very foundations. Though somewhat dense, the book is a seminal work which sets the context for the way in which caring for breech babies may have evolved quite separately from the available research evidence.

Wolf, Naomi (2001) *Misconceptions: Truth, Lies and the Unexpected on the Journey to Motherhood*. Chatto and Windus, London. ISBN 0–7011–6727–0
The first part of this book is a very personal account of a well-known feminist author's journey through her first pregnancy and birth. Although it describes an American obstetric system with all its differences to the UK, much of her disappointment and disillusion felt all too familiar. Her feminist analysis provides useful illumination of the process of pregnancy.

References

1. Abrams, I.F., Bresnan, M.J. and Zuckerman, J.E. (1976) Cervical cord injuries secondary to hyperextension of the head in breech presentation. *Obstetrics and Gynaecology* 41: 369

2. Abu-Heija, A.T., Ziadeh, S. and Obeidat, A. (1997) Breech delivery at term: do the perinatal results justify a trial of labour? *Journal of Obstetrics and Gynaecology* 17(3): 258–60

3. Acien, P. (1993) Reproductive performance of women with uterine malformations. *Human Reproduction* 8: 122–6

4. Acien, P. (1995) Breech presentation in Spain in 1992: a collaborative study. *European Journal of Obstetrics and Gynaecology and Reproductive Biology* 62: 19–24

5. Acien, P. (1996) A comparative study on breech deliveries attended in 1992: hospital centres from Latin America, United States, Spain and Portugal. *European Journal of Obstetrics and Gynaecology and Reproductive Biology* 67: 9–15

6. Albrechtson, S., Rasmussen, S., Dalaker, K. and Irgens, L.M. (1998) Perinatal mortality in breech presentation sibships. *Obstetrics and Gynaecology* 92(5): 775–80

7. Albrechtson, S., Rasmussen, S., Reigstad, H., Markestad, T., Irgens, L.M. and Dalaker, K. (1997) Evaluation of a protocol for selecting fetuses in breech presentation for vaginal delivery or caesarean section. *American Journal of Obstetrics and Gynecology* 177: 586–92

8. Ambadekar, N.N., Khandait, D.W., Sodpey, S.P., Kasturwar, N.B. and Vasude, N.D. (1999) Teenage pregnancy outcome: a record based study. *Indian Journal of Medical Science* 53(1): 14–17

9. Ameghino, J. (1999) Once more out of the breech. *Guardian*, 22 June, p14

10. American College of Obstetricians and Gynaecologists (1997) External cephalic version. *International Journal of Obstetrics and Gynaecology* 59: 73–80

11. Amon, E., Sibai, B.M. and Anderson, G.D. (1988) How perinatologists manage the problem of the presenting breech. *American Journal of Perinatology* 5(3): 247–50

12. Annual Statistical Return Report (1993) Royal College of Obstetricians and Gynaecologists, London

13. Arulkumaran, S., Skurr, B., Tong, H., Kek, L.P. and Ratnam, S.S. (1991) No evidence of hearing loss due to acoustic stimulation test. *Obstetrics and Gynaecology* 78: 283–5

14. Balaskas, J. (1989) *New Active Birth.* Thorsons, London

15. Ballas, S., Toaff, R. and Jaffa, A.J. (1978) Deflexion of the fetal head in breech presentation: incidence, management and outcome. *Obstetrics and Gynaecology* 52: 653

16. Banks, M. (1998) *Breech Birth Woman-Wise.* Birthspirit Books, Hamilton, New Zealand

17. Banks, M. (1996) Breech Birth Woman-Wise. *New Zealand College of Midwives Journal* 15: 17–19

18. Barlov, K. and Larsson, G. (1986) Results of a five year prospective study using a feto-pelvic scoring system for term singleton breech delivery after uncomplicated pregnancy. *Acta Obstetricia Gynecologica Scandinavica* 65: 315–19

19. Bartlett, D. and Okun, N. (1994) Breech presentation: a random event or an explainable phenomenon? *Developmental Medicine and Child Neurology* 36: 833–8

20. Bartlett, D.J., Okun, N.B., Byrne, P.J., Watt, J.M. and Piper, M.C. (2000) Early motor development of breech and cephalic presentation infants. *Obstetrics and Gynaecology* 95(3): 425–32

21. Bartlett, D., Piper, M., Okun, N., Byrne, P. and Watt, J. (1997) Primitive reflexes and the determination of fetal presentation at birth. *Early Human Development* 48(3): 261–73

22. Benifla, J.L., Goffinet, F., Darai, E., et al. (1994) Antepartum transabdominal amnioinfusion to facilitate external cephalic version after initial failure. *Obstetrics and Gynaecology* 84(6): 1041–2

23. Bennebroek Gravenhorst, J., Schreuder, A.M., Veen, S., Brand, R., Verloove-Vanhorick, S.P., Verweij, R.A., Van Zeben van der Aa, D.M. and Ens Dokkum, M.H. (1993) Breech delivery in very preterm and very low birthweight infants in the Netherlands. *British Journal of Obstetrics and Gynaecology* 100: 411–15

24. Ben-Rafael, Z., Seidmena, D.S., Recabi, K., Bider, D. and Mashiach, S. (1991) Uterine anomalies: a retrospective matched-control study. *Journal of Reproductive Medicine* 36: 723–7

25. Berendes, H.W., Weiss, W., Deutschberger, J. and Jackson, E. (1965) Factors associated with breech delivery. *American Journal of Public Health* 55: 708–19

26. Bergstrom, S. (1992) External cephalic version and daily post versional maternal assessment of fetal presentation: a prospective study. *Gynaecological and Obstetric Investigations* 33: 15–18

27. Bewley, S. (1992) Outcome of breech delivery at term. *British Medical Journal* 305: 1499

28. Bewley, S., Robson, S.C., Smith, M., Glover, A. and Spencer, J.A. (1993) The introduction of external cephalic version at term into routine clinical practice. *European Journal of Obstetrics, Gynaecology and Reproductive Biology* 52: 89–93

29. Bilodeau, R. and Marier, R. (1978) Breech presentation at term. *American Journal of Obstetrics and Gynecology* 130: 555–7

30. Bingham, P. and Lilford, R.J. (1987) Management of the selected term breech presentation: assessment of the risks of selected vaginal breech delivery versus caesarean section for all cases. *Obstetrics and Gynaecology* 69: 965–78

30a. Biswas, A. Letter to the Editor. *Lancet* 357 (9251): 225

31. Biswas, A. and Johnstone, M.J. (1993) Term breech delivery: does X-ray pelvimetry help? *Australian and New Zealand Journal of Obstetrics and Gynaecology* 33(2): 150–3

32. Bock, J.E. (1969) The influence of prophylactic external cephalic version on the incidence of breech delivery. A retrospective study. *Acta Obstetricia Gynecologica Scandinavica* 48: 215–21

33. Bradley-Watson, P.J. (1975) The decreasing value of external cephalic version in modern obstetric practice. *American Journal of Obstetrics and Gynecology* 123: 237–40

34. Brenner, W.E., Bruce, R.D. and Hendricks, C.H. (1974) The characteristics and perils of breech presentation. *American Journal of Obstetrics and Gynecology* 118: 700–12

35. Brocks, V., Philipsen, T. and Secher, N.J. (1984) A randomized trial of external cephalic versions with tocolysis in late pregnancy. *British Journal of Obstetrics and Gynaecology* 91: 653–6

36. Brown, L., Karrison, T. and Cibils, L.A. (1994) Mode of delivery and perinatal results in breech presentation. *British Journal of Obstetrics and Gynaecology* 171(1): 28–34

37. Bulfin, M.J. and Gallagher, J.T. (1960) The primipara with breech presentation. *Obstetrics and Gynaecology* 16: 283–7

38. Calhoun, B.C., Edgeworth, D. and Brehm, W. (1995) External cephalic version at a military teaching hospital: predictors of success. *Australian and New Zealand Journal of Obstetrics and Gynaecology* 35: 277–9

39. Campbell, R. and MacFarlane, A. (1987) *Where to be Born?* Oxford National Perinatal Epidemiology Unit, Oxford.

40. Cardini, F., Basevi, V., Valentinie, A. and Martellato, A. (1991) Moxibustion and breech presentation. *American Journal of Chinese Medicine* XIX(2): 105–14

41. Cardozo, I.D. and Kelleher, C.J. (1992) Outcome of breech delivery at term. *British Medical Journal* 305: 1090–1

42. Carlan, S.J., Dent, J.M., Huckaby, T., Whittington, E.C. and Shaefer, D. (1994) The effect of epidural anaesthesia on safety and success of external cephalic version at term. *Anaesthesia and Analgesia* 79: 525–8

43. Cartledge, L.J. and Hancock, F.Y. (1942) Inherited breech presentation. *Journal of Heredity* 33: 409–10

44. Caseaux, P. and Tarnier, S. (1885) *Obstetrics: The Theory and Practice* (ed. Hess, R.J.). 7th edition. London

45. Caterini, H., Langer, A. and Sama, J.C. (1975) Fetal risk in hyperextension of the fetal head in breech presentation. *American Journal of Obstetrics and Gynecology* 123: 632

46. Catt, A. (1997) Sadie's Birth. *New Generation*, 12–13 March

47. Chadha, Y.C., Mahmood, T.A., Dick, M.J., Smith, N.C., Campbell, D.M. and Templeton, A. (1992) Breech delivery and epidural analgesia. *British Journal of Obstetrics and Gynaecology* 99: 96–100

48. Cheek, D. and Rossi, E. (1989) *Mind–Body Hypnosis*. W.W. Norton and Co., New York

49. Cheng, M. and Hannah, M. (1993) Breech delivery at term: a critical review of the literature. *Obstetrics and Gynaecology* 82(4): 605–18

50. Chenia, F. and Crowther, C.A. (1987) Does advice to assume the knee-chest position reduce the incidence of breech presentation at delivery? A randomised clinical trial. *Birth* 14(2): 75–8

51. Chestnut, D.H., Laszewski, L.J., Pollack, K.L., et al. (1990) Continuous epidural infusion of 0.0625% bupivacaine – 0.0002% fentanyl during the second stage of labour. *Anesthesiology* 72(4): 613–18

52. Chestnut, D.H., Vandewalker, G.E., Owen, C.L., et al. (1987) The influence of continuous epidural bupivacaine analgesia on the second stage of labour and method of delivery in nulliparous women. *Anesthesiology* 66(6): 774–80

53. Christian, S.S., Brady, K., Read, J.A. and Kopelman, J.N. (1990) Vaginal breech delivery: a five year prospective evaluation of a protocol using computed tomographic pelvimetry. *American Journal of Obstetrics and Gynecology* 163(3): 848–54

54. Chung, T., Neale, E., Lau, T.K. and Rogers, M. (1996) A randomized double blind trial of tocolysis to assist external cephalic version in late pregnancy. *Acta Obstetricia et Gynecologica Scandinavica* 75: 720–4

55. Cibils, L.A., Karrison, T. and Brown, L. (1994) Factors influencing neonatal outcomes in the very low birth weight fetus (<1500 grams) with a breech presentation. *American Journal of Obstetrics and Gynecology* 171(1): 35–42

56. Clark, G.B. (1995) Uterine rotation following attempted external cephalic version. *The Female Patient* 20: 21–4

57. Clay, L.S., Criss, K. and Jackson, U.C. (1993) External cephalic version. *Journal of Nurse Midwifery* 38(2) (Supplement): 72S–79S

58. Clusker, Paul (2000) Personal communication

59. Cockburn, J., Foong, C., Cockburn, P. (1994) Undiagnosed breeches presenting in labour – should they be allowed a trial of labour? *Journal of Obstetrics and Gynaecology* 14: 151–6

60. Collea, J.V., Chein, C. and Quiligan, E.J. (1980) The randomized management of term frank breech presentation: a study of 208 cases. *American Journal of Obstetrics and Gynecology* 137: 208

61. Collis, R.E., Baxandall, M.L., Srikantharajah, I.D., et al. (1994) Combined spinal epidural (CSE) analgesia: technique, management and outcome of 300 mothers. *International Journal of Obstetric Anaesthesiology* 3(2): 75–81

62. Collis, R.E., Davies, D.W.L. and Aveling, W. (1995) Randomized comparison of combined spinal epidural and standard epidural analgesia in labour. *Lancet* 345 (8962): 1413–16

63. Coltart, T., Edmonds, D. K. and Al-Mufti, R. (1997) External Cephalic Version at term: a survey of consultant obstetric practice in the United Kingdom and Republic of Ireland. *British Journal of Obstetrics and Gynaecology* 104: 544–7

64. Confidential Enquiry into Stillbirths and Deaths in Infancy. Executive Summary of the 7th Annual Report. Maternal and Child Health Research Consortium. June 2000.

65. Confino, E., Gleicher, N., Elrad, H., Isajovich, B. and David, M.P. (1985) The breech dilemma: a review. *Obstetric and Gynaecological Survey* 4(6): 330–7

66. Cook, H.A. (1993) Experience with external cephalic version and selective vaginal breech delivery in private practice. *American Journal of Obstetrics and Gynecology* 168(6): 1886–9

67. Cooperative Research Group of Moxibustion Version of Jangxi Province (1980) *Studies of Version by Moxibustion on Zhiyin Points. Research on Acupuncture, Moxibustion and Acupuncture Anaesthesia.* Science Press, Beijing, pp810, B19.

68. Cooperative Research Group of Moxibustion Version of Jangxi Province (1984) Further studies on the clinical effects and the mechanism of version by moxibustion. The Second National Symposium on Acupuncture, Moxibustion and Acupuncture Anaesthesia – Abstracts pp150–1. All China Society of Acupuncture and Moxibustion, Beijing.

69.   Coyle, Alice (2001) Personal communication
70.   Cronk, Mary (2001) Personal communication
71.   Cronk, M. (1998) Keep your hands off the breech. *AIMS Journal* 10(3): 6–9
72.   Croughan-Minihane, M.S., Petitti, D.B., Gordis, L. and Golditch, I. (1990) Morbidity among breech infants according to method of delivery. *Obstetrics and Gynaecology* 75: 821
72a. Cunha-Filho, J.S. and Passos, E.P. (2001) Letter to the Editor. *Lancet* 357 (9251): 225
73.   Da Cruz, V. (1969) *Baillieres Midwives' Dictionary*. Bailliere, Tindall and Cassell, London
74.   Danforth, D.N. and Ellis, A. (1963) Midforceps delivery – a vanishing art. *American Journal of Obstetrics and Gynecology* 86: 29
75.   Daniel, Y., Fait, G., Lessing, J.B., Jaffa, A., David, M.P. and Kupferminc, M.J. (1998) Outcome of 496 term single to breech deliveries in a tertiary center. *American Journal of Perinatology* 15(2): 97–101
76.   Danielian, P.J., Wang, J. and Hall, M.H. (1996) Long term outcome by method of delivery of fetuses in breech presentation at term: population based follow-up. *British Medical Journal* 312: 1451–3
77.   Deans, A.C., Allman, A.C.J. and Steer, P.J. (1992) Outcome of breech delivery at term. *British Medical Journal* 305: 1091
78.   De Leeuw, J.P. (1987) Management of breech presentation in two university hospitals: preliminary results of a prospective comparative study. *European Journal of Obstetrics, Gynaecology and Reproductive Biology* 24: 93–103
79.   De Leeuw, J.P., de Haan, J., Derom, R., Thiery, M., van Maele, G. and Martens, G. (1998) Indications for caesarean section in breech presentation. *European Journal of Obstetrics, Gynaecology and Reproductive Biology* 79: 131–7
80.   De Meeus, J.B., Ellia, F. and Magnin, G. (1998) External cephalic version after previous caesarean section: as series of 38 cases. *European Journal of Obstetrics, Gynaecology and Reproductive Biology* 81(1): 65–8
81.   Deschacht, S. (1999) High risk deliveries underwater. In De Smedt, Y. (ed.) *Waterbirth in the 21st Century*. Fotos, Fabien Raes and VZW Aquarius, Oostende, Belgium
82.   De Smedt, Y. (ed.) (1999) *Waterbirth in the 21st Century*. Fotos, Fabien Raes and VZW Aquarius, Oostende, Belgium
82a. Department of Health (1993) *Changing Childbirth Part One*. Report of the Expert Maternity Group. HMSO, London
83.   Donald, W.L. and Barton, J.J. (1990) Ultrasonography and external cephalic version at term. *American Journal of Obstetrics and Gynecology* 162: 1542–7
84.   Dugoff, L., Stamm, C.A., Jones, O.W. III, Mohling, S.I. and Hawkins, J.L. (1999) The effect of spinal anaesthesia on the success rate of external cephalic version: a randomized trial. *Obstetrics and Gynaecology* 93(3): 345–9
85.   Dunn, P.M. (1976) Maternal and Fetal Aetiological Factors. 5th European Congress of Perinatal Medicine, pp76–81. Uppsala, Sweden, 9–12 June.
86.   Dyson, D.C., Ferguson, J.E. II and Hensleigh, P. (1986) Antepartum external cephalic version under tocolysis. *Obstetrics and Gynaecology* 67: 63–8
87.   Effer, S.B., Saigal, S., Rand, C., Hunter, D.J.S., Stoskopf, B., Harper, A.C., Nimrod, C. and Milner, R. (1983) Effect of delivery method on outcomes in the very low birth weight breech infant: is the improved survival related to caesarean section or other perinatal care manoeuvres? *American Journal of Obstetrics and Gynecology* 145: 123
88.   Eisenberg, D. and Wright, T.L. (1986) *Encounters with Qi. Exploring Chinese Medicine.* Jonathan Cape, London
89.   Eldering, G. and Selke, K. (1999) Water birth – a possible mode of delivery? In De Smedt, Y. (ed.) *Waterbirth in the 21st Century*. Fotos, Fabien Raes and VZW Aquarius, Oostende, Belgium
89a. Elkins, V.H. (1980) "Procedure for turning breech" Personal communication in Enkin, M. and Chalmers, I. (1982) *Effectiveness and Satisfaction in Antenatal Care.* William Heinemann Medical Books Ltd, London
90.   Eller, D.P. and VanDorsten, J.P. (1995) Route of delivery for the breech presentation: a conundrum. *American Journal of Obstetrics and Gynecology* 173(2): 393–8

91.   Emembolu, J. (1992) The preterm breech delivery in Zaria, Northern Nigeria. *International Journal of Gynaecology and Obstetrics* 38: 287–91

92.   Enkin, M., Keirse, M.J.N., Renfrew, M. and James, N. (1995) *A Guide to Effective Care in Pregnancy and Childbirth*, 2nd edition. Oxford University Press, Oxford

93.   Erkaya, S., Tuncer, R.A., Kutlar, I., et al. (1997) Outcome of 1040 consecutive breech deliveries: clinical experience of a maternity hospital in Turkey. *International Journal of Gynaecology and Obstetrics* 59(2): 115–18

93a. Erskine, J. (2001) Letter to the Editor. *Lancet* 357 (9251): 225

94.   Evans, Jane (2001) Personal communication

94a. Eyraud, J.L., Rietmuller, D., Clainquart, N., Schaal, J.P. and Maillet, R. (1997) Is the Mauriceau Manoeuvre deleterious? Study of 103 cases. *Journal of Gynaecology, Obstetrics and Reproductive Biology* (Paris) 26(4): 413–17

95.   Faber-Nijholt, R. (1981) Breech presentation and neurologic morbidity. A comparative study. PhD thesis, University of Groningen, The Netherlands.

96.   Fait, G., Daniel, Y., Lessing, J.B., et al. (1998) Breech delivery: the value of X-ray pelvimetry. *European Journal of Gynaecology, Obstetrics and Reproductive Biology* 78(1): 1–4

97.   Faundes, A. (2001) The risk of urinary incontinence of parous women who delivered only by caesarean section. *International Journal of Gynaecology and Obstetrics* 72: 41–6

98.   Ferguson, J.E., Armstrong, M.A. and Dyson, D.C. (1987) Maternal and fetal factors affecting success of antepartum external cephalic version. *Obstetrics and Gynaecology* 70: 722–5

99.   Ferguson, J.E. II and Dyson, D. (1985) Intrapartum external cephalic version. *American Journal of Obstetrics and Gynecology* 152: 297–8

100. Fianu, S. and Vaclavinkova, V. (1978) The site of placental attachment as a factor in the aetiology of breech presentation. *Acta Obstetricia et Gynaecologica Scandinavica* 57: 371–2

101. Flamm, B.L., Fried, M.W., Lonky, N.M. and Saurenman, G.W. (1991) External cephalic version after previous caesarean section. *American Journal of Obstetrics and Gynecology* 165(2): 370–2

102. Flanagan, T., Mulchahey, K., Korenbrot, C., et al. (1987) Management of term breech presentation. *American Journal of Obstetrics and Gynecology* 156: 1492

103. Flint, Caroline (2000) Personal communication

104. Flint, C. (1986) *Sensitive Midwifery*. Heinemann, Oxford

105. Flint, C. (1989) Babies presenting by the breech. *Obstetric and Gynaecological Product News* (Summer): 21–3

106. Floberg, J., Belfrage, P., Carlsson, M. and Ohlsen, M. (1986) The pelvic outlet. A comparison between clinical evaluation and radiological pelvimetry. *Acta Obstetricia et Gynecologica Scandinavica* 65: 321–6

107. Fortney, J.A., Higgins, J.E., Kennedy, K.I., Laufe, L.E. and Wilkins, L. (1986) Delivery type and neonatal mortality among 10749 breeches. *American Journal of Public Health* 76: 980–5

108. Fortunato, S.J., Mercer, L.J. and Guzick, D.S. (1988) External cephalic version with tocolysis: factors associated with success. *Obstetrics and Gynaecology* 72: 59–62

108a. Francis, Annie (2001) Personal communication

109. Francome, C., Savage, W., Churchill, H. and Lewison, H. (1993) *Caesarean Birth in Britain*. Middlesex University Press, London

110. Friedlander, D. (1996) External cephalic version in the management of breech presentation. A report on 706 patients treated by this method. *American Journal of Obstetrics and Gynecology* 95: 906

111. Garrey, M.M., Govan, A.D.T., Hodge, C. and Callander, R. (1974) *Obstetrics Illustrated*. Churchill Livingstone, Edinburgh and London

112. Gaskin, I.M. (1994) Statistics for 1888 births attended by the Farm midwives November 1970 – April 1994. *Birth Gazette* (Summer)

113. Gaskin, I.M. (1990) *Spiritual Midwifery*. Book Publishing Company, Summertown, Tennessee

114. Geutjens, G., Gilbert, A. and Helson, K. (1996) Obstetric Brachial Plexus Palsy associated with breech delivery. *Journal of Bone and Joint Surgery* 78-B(2) (March): 303–6

115. Gibb, Donald (2000) Personal communication

116. Gilady, Y., Battino, S., Reich, D., Gilad, G. and Shalev, E. (1996) Delivery of the very low birthweight breech: what is the best way for the baby? *Israel Journal of Medical Science* 32(2): 116–20

117. Gimovsky, M.L. and Petrie, R.H. (1982) Management of the breech presentation. *Perinatology and Neonatology* 6: 73–8

118. Gimovsky, M.L. and Schifrin, M. (1992) Breech management. *Journal of Perinatology* 12: 143–51

119. Gimovsky, M.L., Wallace, R.L., Schifrin, B.S. and Paul, R.H. (1983) Randomized management of the nonfrank breech presentation at term: a preliminary report. *American Journal of Obstetrics and Gynecology* 146: 34

120. Gjode, P., Rasmussen, T.B. and Jorgensen, J. (1980) Feto-maternal bleeding during attempts at external cephalic version. *British Journal of Obstetrics and Gynaecology* 87: 571–3

120a. Goethals, T.R. (1956) Caesarean section as the method of choice in management of breech delivery. *American Journal of Obstetrics and Gynecology* 71: 536

121. Goh, J.T., Johnson, C.M. and Gregora, M.G. (1993) External cephalic version at term. *Australian and New Zealand Journal of Obstetrics and Gynaecology* 33: 364–6

122. Gorbe, E., Hajdu, J., Harmath, A., Sztanyik, L. and Papp, Z. (1997) The effect of the delivery method on the mortality of very low birth weight infants in case of breech presentation. *Orv Hetil* 138(24): 1561–4

123. Gordon, Yehudi (2000) Personal communication

124. Green, J.E., McLean, F., Smith, L.P. and Usher, R. (1982) Has an increased caesarean section rate for term breech delivery reduced the incidence of birth asphyxia, trauma and death? *American Journal of Obstetrics and Gynecology* 142: 643–8

125. Hall, M. and Bewley, S. (1999) Maternal mortality and mode of delivery. *Lancet* 354: 776

126. Hannah, M. and Hannah, W. (1996) Caesarean section or vaginal birth for breech presentation at term. *British Medical Journal* 312: 1433

127. Hannah, M.E., Hannah, W.J., Hewson, S.A., Hodnett, E.D., Saigal, S. and Willan, A.R. (2000) Planned caesarean section versus planned vaginal birth for breech presentation at term: a randomised multicentre trial. *Lancet* 356: 1375–83

128. Hawkey, M. (1997) Acupuncture: an alternative option in pregnancy. *British Journal of Midwifery* 5(7): 559

129. Healey, M., Porter, R. and Galimberti, A. (1997) Introducing external cephalic version at 36 weeks or more in a district general hospital: a review and an audit. *British Journal of Obstetrics and Gynaecology* 104: 1073–9

130. Helfferich, M. and Favier, J. (1971) Breech delivery. *American Journal of Obstetrics and Gynecology* 110(1): 58–61

131. Hellstrom, A.C., Nilsson, B., Stange, L. and Nyland, L. (1990) When does external cephalic version succeed? *Acta Obstetricia et Gynecologica Scandinavica* 69: 281–5

132. Hickock, D., Gordon, D., Milberg, J., et al. (1992) The frequency of breech presentation by gestational age at term: a large population based study. *American Journal of Obstetrics and Gynecology* 166: 851

133. Hill, L. (1990) Prevalence of breech presentation by gestational age. *American Journal of Perinatology* 7: 92

134. Hofmeyr, G.J. (1983) Effect of external cephalic version in late pregnancy on breech presentation and caesarean section rate: a controlled trial. *British Journal of Obstetrics and Gynaecology* 90: 392–9

135. Hofmeyr, G.J. (1998) External cephalic version at term. (Cochrane review). In *The Cochrane Library*, Issue 2, Oxford. Update software; 1998. Updated quarterly

136. Hofmeyr, G.J. and Hannah, M.E. (2001) Planned caesarean section for term breech delivery (review). Cochrane Database Systematic Review 1 CD000166

137. Hofmeyr, G.J., Sadan, O., Myer, I.G., Galal, K.C. and Simko, G. (1986) External cephalic version and spontaneous version rates: ethnic and other determinants. *British Journal of Obstetrics and Gynaecology* 93(1): 13–16

138. Howell, C.J. (1995) Epidural vs non-epidural anaesthesia in labour [revised 06 May 1994]. In Keirse, M.J.N.C., Renfrew, M.J., Neilson, J.P. and Crowther, C. (eds) *Pregnancy and Childbirth*

Module. In: *The Cochrane Pregnancy and Childbirth Database, The Cochrane Collaboration: Issue 2,* Oxford: Update software 1995. BMJ publishing group, London

139. Hughes, G.W. (1998) The value of external cephalic version. *Contemporary Reviews in Obstetrics and Gynaecology* (June): 91–8

140. Huntingford, P. (1985) *Birth Right – The Parent's Choice.* British Broadcasting Corporation, London.

141. Impey, L. and Lissoni, D. (1999) Outcome of external cephalic version after 36 weeks gestation without tocolysis. *Journal of Maternal and Fetal Medicine* 8(5): 203–7

141a. Iovine, V. (1997) *The Best Friend's Guide to Pregnancy.* Bloomsbury, London

142. Irion, O., Hirsbrunner Almagbaly, P. and Morabia, A. (1998) Planned vaginal delivery versus elective caesarean section: a study of 705 singleton term breech presentations. *British Journal of Obstetrics and Gynaecology* 105: 710–7

143. Ismail, M.A., Nagib, N., Ismail, T. and Cibils, L.A. (1999) Comparison of vaginal and cesarean section delivery for fetuses in breech presentation. *Journal of Perinatal Medicine* 5: 339–51

144. Jaffa, A.J., Peyser, M.R., Ballas, S. and Toaff, R. (1981) Management of term breech presentation in primigravidae. *British Journal of Obstetrics and Gynaecology* 88: 721

145. Johanson, R. (1998) External cephalic version. *The Diplomate* 5(3): 178–82

146. Johnson, R.L. and Elliott, J.P. (1995) Fetal acoustic stimulation, an adjunct to external cephalic version: a blinded randomized crossover study. *American Journal of Obstetrics and Gynecology* 173(5): 1369–72

147. Johnson, R.L., Strong, T.H. Jr, Radin, T. and Elliott, J.P. (1995) Fetal acoustic stimulation as an adjunct to external version. *Journal of Reproductive Medicine* 40(10): 1369–72

148. Jolly, J., Walker, J. and Bhabra, K. (1999) Subsequent obstetric performance related to primary mode of delivery. *British Journal of Obstetrics and Gynaecology* 106: 227–32

149. Karp, L.E. (1983) Breech presentation and parity: the proof of the pelvis. *Journal of the American Medical Association* 249(5): 647

150. Kasule, J., Chimbira, T.H. and Brown, I.M. (1985) Controlled trial of external cephalic version. *British Journal of Obstetrics and Gynaecology* 92: 14–18

151. Kauppila, O. (1975) The perinatal mortality in breech deliveries and observations on affecting factors: a retrospective study on 2227 cases. *Acta Obstetricia et Gynecologica Scandinavica* (Supplement) 39: 1–79

152. Kean, L.H., Suwanrath, C., Gargari, S.S., Sahota, D.S. and James, D.K. (1999) A comparison of fetal behaviour in breech and cephalic presentations at term. *British Journal of Obstetrics and Gynaecology* 106(11): 1209–13

153. Kiely, J.L. (1991) Mode of delivery and neonatal death in 17587 infants presenting by the breech. *British Journal of Obstetrics and Gynaecology* 98: 898–904

154. Kian L.S. (1963) The role of placental site in the aetiology of breech presentation. A clinical survey of 362 cases. *Journal of Obstetrics and Gynaecology of the British Commonwealth* 70: 795–7

155. Kingdom, J. and Murphy, K. (1992) Outcome of breech delivery at term. *British Medical Journal* 305: 1090

155a. Kitzinger, S. (1987) *Freedom and Choice in Childbirth.* Penguin, London

156. Kitzinger, S. (1990) *Episiotomy and the Second Stage of Labour.* Penny Press, London

157. Koo, M.R., Dekker, G.A. and van Geijn, H.P. (1998) Perinatal outcome of singleton term breech deliveries. *European Journal of Obstetrics, Gynaecology and Reproductive Biology* 78(1): 19–24

158. Korte, D. and Scaer, R. (1992) *A Good Birth – A Safe Birth.* Harvard Common Press, Boston

159. Kott, Barbara (2001) Personal communication

160. Krebs, L., Langhoff-Roos, J. and Weber, T. (1995) Breech at term – mode of delivery? *Acta Obstetricia et Gynecologica Scandinavica* 74: 702–6

161. Krebs, L., Topp, M. and Langhoff-Roos, J. (1999) The relation of breech presentation at term to cerebral palsy. *British Journal of Obstetrics and Gynaecology* 106(9): 943–7

163. Kunzel, W. (1995) Recommendations of the FIGO Committee on Perinatal Health on guidelines for the management of breech delivery. *European Journal of Obstetrics, Gynaecology and Reproductive Biology* 58: 89–92

163a. Lagercrantz, H. and Slotkin, T.A. (1986) The "stress" of being born. *Scientific American* 254(4): 92–107

164. Langer, B., Boudier, E. and Schlaeder, G. (1998) Breech presentation after 34 weeks – a meta-analysis of corrected perinatal mortality/morbidity according to the method of delivery. *Journal of Obstetrics and Gynaecology* 18: 127–32

165. Lau, T.K., Stock, A. and Rogers, M. (1995) Fetomaternal haemorrhage after external cephalic version at term. *Australian and New Zealand Journal of Obstetrics and Gynaecology* 35: 173–4

166. Lau, K.T., Lo, K.W.K., Wan, D. and Rogers, M. (1997) Predictors of successful external cephalic version at term: a prospective study. *British Journal of Obstetrics and Gynaecology* 104: 798–802

167. Lavin, J., et al. (1982) Vaginal delivery in patients with a prior caesarean section. *Obstetrics and Gynaecology* 59: 135

168. Law, R.G. (1967) *Standards of Obstetric Care. The report of the north-west metropolitan regional obstetric survey 1962–4.* Livingstone, Edinburgh, pp10–89

169. Lee, K.S., Khoshnood, B., Sriram, S., Hsieh, H.L., Singh, J. and Mittendorf, R. (1998) Relationship of caesarean delivery to lower birth weight specific neonatal mortality in singleton breech infants in the United States. *Obstetrics and Gynaecology* 92(5): 769–74

170. Lennox, C.E., Kwast, B.E. and Farley, T.M.M. (1998) Breech labor on the WHO partograph. *International Journal of Obstetrics and Gynaecology* 62: 117–27

171. Leung, W.C., Pun, T.C. and Wong, W.M. (1999) Undiagnosed breech revisited. *British Journal of Obstetrics and Gynaecology* 106(7): 638–41

172. Levine, E.M., Ghai, V., Barton, J.J. and Strom, C.M. (2001) Mode of delivery and risk of respiratory diseases in newborns. *Obstetrics and Gynaecology* 97: 439–42

173. Lilford, R.J., Van Coeverden de Groot, H.A., Moore, P.J. and Bingham, P. (1990) The relative risks of caesarean section (intrapartum and elective) and vaginal delivery: a detailed analysis to exclude the effects of medical disorders and other acute pre-existing physiological disturbances. *British Journal of Obstetrics and Gynaecology* 97: 883–92

174. Lindqvist, A., Norden-Lindeberg, S. and Hanson, U. (1997) Perinatal mortality and route of delivery in term breech presentations. *British Journal of Obstetrics and Gynaecology* 104: 1288–91

175. Lowden G. (1998) Natural active breech birth. *Aims Journal* 10:(3) 5

176. Lowden, G. (1998) Why are some babies breech? *Aims Journal* 10(3): 8–9

177. Lumley, J. (2000) Any room left for disagreement about assisting breech births at term? *Lancet* 356 (21 October): 368–9

178. Luterkort, M., Persson, P. and Weldner, B. (1984) Maternal and fetal factors in breech presentation. *Obstetrics and Gynaecology* 64(1) (June): 55–9

179. Machover, I. (1995) Turn, baby, turn. *Midwives* (November)

180. Mackenzie, I.Z. and Jefferies, M. (1992) Outcome of breech delivery at term. *British Medical Journal* 305: 1499

181. Mahomed, K., Seeras, R. and Coulson, R. (1991) External cephalic version at term. A randomized controlled trial using tocolysis. *British Journal of Obstetrics and Gynaecology* 98: 8–13

182. Makris, N., Xygakis, A., Chionism, A., Sakellaropoulos, G. and Michalas, S. (1999) The management of breech presentation in the last three decades. *Clinical Experimental Obstetrics and Gynaecology* 26(3–4): 178–80

183. Malhotra, D., Gopalan, S. and Narang, A. (1994) Preterm breech delivery in a developing country. *International Journal of Obstetrics and Gynaecology* 45: 27–34

184. Marchick, R. (1988) Antepartum external cephalic version with tocolysis: a study of term singleton breech presentations. *American Journal of Obstetrics and Gynecology* 158: 1339–46

185. Marquette, G.P., Boucher, M., Theriault, D. and Rinfret, D. (1996) Does the use of a tocolytic agent affect the success rate of external cephalic version? *American Journal of Obstetrics and Gynecology* 175: 859–61

186. Marsden, W. (2000) Choosing caesarean section. *Lancet* 356: 1677–80

187.   Mauldin, J.G., Mauldin, P.D., Feng, T.I., Adams, E.K. and Durkalski, V.L. (1996) Determining the clinical efficacy and cost savings of successful external cephalic version. *American Journal of Obstetrics and Gynecology* 175(6): 1639–44

188.   Mayank, S. and Kripilani, A. (1997) Fetal demise following external cephalic version. *International Journal of Gynaecology and Obstetrics* 56(2): 177–8

189.   McParland, P. and Farine, D. (1996) External cephalic version: does it have a role in modern obstetric practice? *Canadian Family Physician* 42: 693–8

190.   Mehl, L.E. (1994) Hypnosis and conversion of the breech to the vertex presentation. *Archives of Family Medicine* (3 October): 881–7

191.   Meniru, G. and Reginald, P.W. (1994) Deeply engaged head: is it a breech presentation? *Journal of Obstetrics and Gynaecology* 14: 256–7

192.   Michalas, S.P. (1991) Outcome of pregnancy in women with uterine malformation: evaluation of 62 cases. *International Journal of Gynaecology and Obstetrics* 35: 215–19

193.   Midirs and the NHS Centre for Reviews and Dissemination (1997) *Breech Baby – Options for Care*. Midirs, Bristol

194.   Midirs and the NHS Centre for Reviews and Dissemination (1997) *Epidural Pain Relief During Labour*. Midirs, Bristol

195.   Midirs and the NHS Centre for Reviews and Dissemination (1997) *Fetal Heart Rate Monitoring in Labour*. Midirs, Bristol

196.   Milner, R.D.G. (1975) Neonatal mortality of breech deliveries with and without forceps to the aftercoming head. *British Journal of Obstetrics and Gynaecology* 82: 783–5

197.   Minogue, M. (1974) Vaginal breech delivery in multiparae – National Maternity Hospital. *Journal of the Irish Medical Association* 67: 117–19

198.   Mitford, J. (1992) *The American Way of Birth*. Victor Gollancz, London

199.   Moore, Tracey (1998) Personal communication

200.   Morgan, H.S. and Kane, S.H. (1964) An analysis of 16327 breech births. *Journal of the American Medical Association* 187: 108–10

201.   Morrison, J.C., Myatt, R.E., Martin, J.N. Jr, Meeks, G.R., Martin, R.W., Bucovaz, E.T., et al. (1986) External cephalic version of the breech presentation under tocolysis. *American Journal of Obstetrics and Gynecology* 154: 900–3

202.   Morton, S.C., Williams, M.S., Keeler, E.B., et al. (1994) Effect of epidural analgesia for labour on the caesarean delivery rate. *Obstetrics and Gynaecology* 83(6): 1045–52

203.   Myerscough, P. (1998) The practice of external cephalic version. *British Journal of Obstetrics and Gynaecology* 105: 1043–5

204.   Nahid, F. (2000) Outcome of singleton term breech cases in the pretext of mode of delivery. *Journal of the Pakistani Medical Association* 50(3): 81–5

205.   Narakas, A.O. (1987) Obstetrical brachial plexus injuries. In Lamb, D.W. (ed.) *The Paralyzed Hand and Upper Limb*, Vol. 2. Churchill Livingstone, Edinburgh, pp116–35

206.   Neil, W.R. (1991) *The Complete Handbook of Pregnancy*. Little Brown and Company, London

207.   Neimand, K. and Rosenthal, A. (1965) Oxytocin in breech presentation. *American Journal of Obstetrics and Gynecology* 93: 230–6

208.   Neri Ruiz, E.S., Valerio Castro, E., Cardenas Arias, R. and Navarro Milla, O. (1997) Pelvic presentation, always a caesarean? *Ginecologia y Obstetricia de Mexico* 65: 474–7

209.   Newman, R.B., Peacock, B.S., Van Dorsten, J.P. and Hunt, H.H. (1993) Predicting the success of external cephalic version. *American Journal of Obstetrics and Gynecology* 169(2)(1): 245–9

210.   Nielson, T.F. and Hokegard, K.H. (1983) Postoperative caesarean section morbidity: a prospective study. *American Journal of Obstetrics and Gynecology* 146: 911–16

211.   Nwosu, E.C., Walkinshaw, S., Chia, P., Manasse, P.R. and Atlay R.D. (1993) Undiagnosed breech. *British Journal of Obstetrics and Gynaecology* 100: 531–5

212.   Odent, Michel (2000) Personal communication

213.   Odent, M. (1984) *Birth Reborn*. Random House, London

214.   Odent, M. (2000) The second stage as a disruption of the fetus ejection reflex. *Midwifery Today* 55: 12

215.   Oian, P., Skramm, I., Hannisdal, E. and Bjoro, K. (1988) Breech delivery: an obstetrical analysis. *Acta Obstetricia et Gynecologica Scandinavica* 67: 75–9

216. O' Leary, J.A. (1979) Vaginal delivery of the term breech. A preliminary report. *Obstetrics and Gynaecology* 53: 341–3

217. Omu, A.E. and Akingba, J.B. (1986) Trends in management of breech presentation in Benin city. *Nigerian Medical Journal* 16: 19–26

218. Ophir, E., Oettinger, M., Yagoda, A., Markovits, Y., Rojansky, N. and Shapiro, H. (1989) Breech presentation after caesarean section: Always a section? *American Journal of Obstetrics and Gynecology* 161(1): 25–8

219. Pajntar, M., Verdenik, I. and Pestevsek, M. (1994) Caesarean section in breech by birth weight. *European Journal of Obstetrics, Gynaecology and Reproductive Biology* 54: 181–4

220. Parsons, M.T. and Spellacy, W.N. (1985) Prospective randomized study of X-ray pelvimetry in the primigravida. *Obstetrics and Gynaecology* 66: 76–9

221. Patek, E. and Larsson, B. (1978) Caesarean section. *Acta Obstetricia et Gynecologica Scandinavica* 57: 245–8

222. Paterson-Brown, S. and Fisk, N.M. (1992) Outcome of breech delivery at term. *British Medical Journal* 305: 1091

223. Peisne, D.B. and Rosen, M.G. (1992) Normal and operative deliveries. In Reece, E.A., Hobbins, J.C., Mahoney, M.J. and Petrie, R.H. (eds) *Medicine of the Fetus and Mother*. J.B. Lippincott Co., Philadelphia, pp1389–90

224. Penkin, P., Cheng, M. and Hannah, M. (1996) Survey of Canadian obstetricians regarding the management of term breech presentation. *Journal of the Society of Obstetricians and Gynaecologists of Canada* (March): 233–42

225. Penn, Z.J. and Steer, P.J. (1991) How obstetricians manage the problem of preterm delivery with special reference to the preterm breech. *British Journal of Obstetrics and Gynaecology* 98 (June): 531–4

226. Penn, Z.J. and Steer, P.J. (1996) A multi-centre randomised controlled trial to compare elective versus selective caesarean section for the delivery of the preterm breech infant. *British Journal of Obstetrics and Gynaecology* 103: 684–9

227. Phelan, J.P., Stine, L.E., Edwards, N.B., Clark, S.L. and Horenstein, J. (1985) The role of external version in the intrapartum management of the transverse lie presentation. *American Journal of Obstetrics and Gynecology* 151: 724–6

228. Philipsen, T. and Jensen, N.H. (1989) Epidural block parenteral pethidine as analgesic in labour: a randomized study concerning progress in labour and instrumental deliveries. *European Journal of Obstetrics, Gynaecology and Reproductive Biology* 30(1): 27–33

229. Plaut, M., Schwartz, M. and Lubarsky, S. (1999) Uterine rupture associated with the use of misoprostol in the gravid patient with a previous caesarean section. *American Journal of Obstetrics and Gynecology* 180: 1535–42

230. Plentl, A.A. and Stone, R.E. (1953) The Bracht Manoeuvre. *Obstetrical and Gynaecological Survey* 8: 313–25

231. Potter, M.G., Heaton, C.E. and Douglas, G.W. (1960) Intrinsic fetal risk in breech delivery. *Obstetrics and Gynaecology* 15: 158–62

231a. Premru-Srxsen, T. (2001) Letter to the Editor. *Lancet* 357 (9251): 225–6

232. Ramin, S.M., Gambling, D.R., Lucas, M.J., et al. (1995) Randomized trial of epidural versus intravenous analgesia during labour. *Obstetrics and Gynaecology* 86(5): 783–9

233. Ranney, B. (1973) The gentle art of external cephalic version. *American Journal of Obstetrics and Gynecology* 116: 239–51

234. Ray, J. (1993) My version. *Birth Gazette* 9(2): 30–1

235. Rayl, J., Gibson, P.J. and Hickok, D.E. (1996) A population based case-control study of risk factors for breech presentation. *American Journal of Obstetrics and Gynecology* 174(1) (January): 28–33

236. RCOG (1993) *The Effective Procedures in Obstetrics Suitable for Audit*. RCOG Audit Unit, Manchester, July.

237. Report of the Expert Maternity Group (1993) *Changing Childbirth*. HMSO, London.

238. Richards, L. Baptisti (1987) *The Vaginal Birth After Caesarean Experience*. Bergin & Garvey, South Hadley, MA

239. Roberts, C.L., Algert, C.S., Peat, B. and Henderson-Smart, D. (1999) Small fetal size: a risk factor for breech birth at term. *International Journal of Obstetrics and Gynaecology* 67(1): 1–8

240. Robertson, A.W., Kopelman, J.N., Read, J.A., Duff, P., Magelsson, D.J. and Dashow, E.E. (1987) External cephalic version at term: is a tocolytic necessary? *Obstetrics and Gynaecology* 70: 896–9

241. Robertson, P.A., Foran, C.M., Croughan-Minihane, M.S. and Kilpatrick, S.J. (1996) Head entrapment and neonatal outcome by mode of delivery in breech deliveries from 28 to 36 weeks of gestation. *American Journal of Obstetrics and Gynecology* 174(6): 1742–9

242. Robinson, Jean (2001) Personal communication

243. Roman, J., Bakos, O. and Cnattingius, S. (1998) Pregnancy outcomes by mode of delivery among term breech births: Swedish experience 1987–93. *Obstetrics and Gynaecology* 92(6): 945–50

244. Rosen, M.G., Debanne, S., Thompson, K. and Bilenker, R.M. (1985) Long term neurological morbidity in breech and vertex births. *American Journal of Obstetrics and Gynecology* 151: 718–23

245. Rovinsky, J.J., Miller, J.A. and Kaplan, S. (1973) Management of breech presentation at term. *American Journal of Obstetrics and Gynecology* 115: 746–7

246. Sachs, B.P., Mccarthy, B.J., Rubin, G., Burton, A., Terry, J. and Tyler, C.W. (1983) Caesarean section: risks and benefits for mother and fetus. *Journal of the American Medical Association* 250(16): 2157–9

247. Saling, E. and Muller-Holve, W. (1975) External cephalic version under tocolysis. *Journal of Perinatal Medicine* 3: 115–22

248. Saunders, N.J. (1996a) Breech delivery in the United Kingdom at the end of this century. *Contemporary Review in Obstetrics and Gynaecology* 8: 82–5

249. Saunders, N.J. (1996b) The management of breech presentation. *British Journal of Hospital Medicine* 56(9): 456–8

250. Saunders, Nigel (2001) Personal communication

251. Savage, W. (1989) The effect of the attitudes of the obstetrician on the birthing woman. In van Hall, E.V. and Everard, W. (eds) *The Free Woman: Women's Health in the 1990s*. Parthenon, Lancashire, UK

252. Savage, Wendy (2000) Personal communication

253. Scaling, S.T. (1988) External cephalic version without tocolysis. *American Journal of Obstetrics and Gynecology* 158: 1424–30

254. Schacter, M., Kogan, S. and Blickstein, I. (1994) External cephalic version after previous caesarean section – a clinical dilemma. *International Journal of Gynaecology and Obstetrics* 45: 17–20

255. Scheer, K. and Nubar, J. (1976) Variation of fetal presentation with gestational age. *American Journal of Obstetrics and Gynecology* 125: 269

256. Schiff, E., Friedman, S.A., Mashiach, S., Hart, O., Barkai, G. and Sibai, B.M. (1996) Maternal and neonatal outcome of 846 term singleton breech deliveries: seven year experience at a single centre. *American Journal of Obstetrics and Gynecology* 175(1): 18–23

257. Schorr, S.J., Speights, S.E., Ross, E.L., Bofill, J.A., Rust, O.A., Norman, P.F. and Morrison, J.C. (1997) A randomized trial of epidural anaesthesia to improve external cephalic version success. *American Journal of Obstetrics and Gynecology* 177(5): 1133–7

258. Schuitemaker, N., van Roosmalen, J., Dekker, G., van Dongen, P., van Geijn, H. and Bennebroek Gravenhorst, J. (1997) Maternal mortality after caesarean section in The Netherlands. *Acta Obstetricia et Gynecologica Scandinavica* 75: 332–4

259. Scorza, W.E. (1996) Intrapartum management of breech presentation. *Clinics in Perinatology* 23(1): 31–49

260. Shalev, E., Battino, S., Giladi, Y. and Edelstien, S. (1993) External cephalic version at term – using tocolysis. *Acta Obstetricia et Gyaecologica Scandinavica* 72: 455–7

261. Sharma, J.B., Newman, M.R., Boutchier, J.E. and Williams, A. (1997) National Audit on the practice and training in breech deliveries in the UK. *International Journal of Gynaecology and Obstetrics* 59: 103–8

262. Shembrey, M.A. and Letchworth, A.T. (1993) The management of breech presentation in a district general hospital. *Journal of Obstetrics and Gynaecology* 13: 437–9

263. Shennan, A. and Bewley, S. (2001) How to manage term breech deliveries. *British Medical Journal* 323: 244–5

264. Siddiqui, D., Stiller, R.J., Collins, J. and Laifer, S.A. (1999) Pregnancy outcome after successful external cephalic version. *American Journal of Obstetrics and Gynecology* 181 5(1): 1092–5

265. Silvert, M. (2000) Doctors need more training in delivering breech babies. *British Medical Journal* 320: 1689

266. Smith, J., Hernandez, C. and Wax, J. (1997) Fetal laceration injury at caesarean delivery. *Obstetrics and Gynaecology* 90: 344–6

267. Smith, J.I. (1978) Caesarean section in management of primigravidas with breech presentations. *Quality Review Bulletin* 4: 16–19

267a. Somerset, D. (2002) Term breech trial does not provide unequivocal evidence. *British Medical Journal* 324 (7328): 49

268. Songane, F., Thobani, S., Malik, H., Bingham, P. and Lilford, R.J. (1987) Balancing the risks of planned caesarean section and trial of vaginal delivery for the mature, selected, singleton breech presentation. *Journal of Perinatal Medicine* 15: 531–4

269. Sorensen, H.T., Steffensen, F.H., Olsen, J., Sabroe, S., Gillman, M.W., Fischer, P. and Rothman, K.J. (1999) Long-term follow-up of cognitive outcome after breech presentation at birth. *Epidemiology* 10(5): 554–6

270. Spelliscy-Gifford, D., Keeler, E. and Kahn, K.L. (1995) Reductions in cost and caesarean rate by routine use of external cephalic version: a decision analysis. *Obstetrics and Gynaecology* 85(6): 930–6

271. Spelliscy-Gifford, D., Morton, S.C., Fiske, M. and Kahn, K. (1995) A meta-analysis of infant outcomes after breech delivery. *Obstetrics and Gynaecology* 85(6): 1047–54

272. Stabler, F. (1947) The cause of polar lie. *Journal of Obstetrics and Gynaecology of the British Empire* 54: 345–450

273. Stein, A. (1986) A cooperative nurse-midwifery medical management approach. *Journal of Nurse Midwifery* 31(2): 93–7

274. Stevenson, C.S. (1950) The principal cause of breech presentation in single term pregnancies. *American Journal of Obstetrics and Gynecology* 60: 41–53

275. Stevenson, C.S. (1951) Certain concepts in the handling of breech and transverse presentations in late pregnancy. *American Journal of Obstetricians and Gynaecologists* 63(3): 488–505

276. Stevenson, J. (1993) More thoughts on breech. *Midwifery Today* 26 (Summer): 24–5

277. Stine, L.E., Phelan, J.P., Wallace, R., Eglinton, G.S., Van Dorsten, J.P. and Schifrin, B.S. (1985) Update on external cephalic version performed at term. *Obstetrics and Gynaecology* 65: 642–6

278. Stock, A., Chung, T., Roger, M. and Ming, W.W. (1993) Randomized double blind controlled comparison of ritodrine and hexoprenaline for tocolysis prior to external cephalic version at term. *Australian and New Zealand Journal of Obstetrics and Gynaecology* 33: 265–8

278a. Stuart, I.P. (2001) Letter to the Editor. *Lancet* 357 (9251): 225

279. Sutton, J. and Scott, P. (1996) *Understanding and Teaching Optimal Foetal Positioning*. Birth Concepts, New Zealand

280. Svenningsen, N.W., Westgren, M. and Ingemarsson, I. (1985) Modern strategy for the term breech delivery: a study with a 4 year follow-up of the infants. *Journal of Perinatal Medicine* 13: 117

281. Swietlicki, F.C. (1995) Breech delivery – the Scottish way of birth. *AIMS Journal* 7(3): 12–14

282. Tan, G.W., Jen, S.W., Tan, S.L. and Salmon, Y.M. (1989) A prospective randomised controlled trial of external cephalic version comparing two methods of uterine tocolysis with a non-tocolysis group. *Singapore Medical Journal* 30: 155–8

283. Taussig, F.J. (1931) Breech presentation. *American Journal of Obstetrics and Gynecology* 22: 304–11

284. Taylor P.J., Hannah, W.J., Allardice, J., et al. (1994) The Canadian consensus on breech management at term. *Journal of the Society of Obstetricians and Gynaecologists of Canada* 16 (June): 1839–48

285. Teoh, T.G. (1997) Effect of learning curve on the outcome of external cephalic version. *Singapore Medical Journal* 38(8): 323–5

286. Tew, M. (1998) *Safer Childbirth? A Critical History of Maternity Care*. Free Association Books, London

287. Thomas, P. (1996) *Every Woman's Birth Rights*. Thorsons, London

288. Thomas, P. (1998) *Choosing a Home Birth*. AIMS, Surbiton

289. Thomas, P. (2000) What's so bad about ultrasound? *Natural Parent* (May/June): 26–8

290. Thornton, J.G. and Lilford, R.J. (1996) Preterm breech babies and randomised trials of rare conditions. *British Journal of Obstetrics and Gynaecology* 103: 611–13

291. Thorp, J.A., Hu, D.H., Albin, R.M., et al. (1993) The effect of intrapartum epidural analgesia on nulliparous labour: a randomised, controlled prospective trial. *American Journal of Obstetrics and Gynecology* 169(4): 851–8

292. Thorp, J.A., Meyer, B.A., Cohen, G.R., et al. (1994) Epidural anaesthesia in labour and caesarean delivery for dystocia. *Obstetric and Gynaecological Survey* 49(5): 362–9

293. Thorpe-Beeston, Guy (2001) Personal communication

294. Thorpe-Beeston, J.G., Banfield, P.J. and Saunders, N.J.St.G. (1992) Outcome of breech delivery at term. *British Medical Journal* 305: 746–7

295. Thunedborg, P., Fischer-Rasmussen, W. and Tollund, L. (1991) The benefit of external cephalic version with tocolysis as a routine procedure in late pregnancy. *European Journal of Obstetrics, Gynaecology and Reproductive Biology* 42: 23–7

296. Todd, W.D. and Steer, C.M. (1963) Tem breech: review of 1006 term breech deliveries. *Obstetrics and Gynaecology* 22: 583–95

297. Tompkins, P. (1946) An inquiry into the causes of breech presentation. *American Journal of Obstetrics and Gynaecology* 51: 595–607

297a. Uchide, K. and Murakami, K. (2001) Letter to the Editor. *Lancet* 357 (9251): 225

298. Van de Pavert, R., Gravenhorst, J.B. and Keirse, M.J.N.C. (1990) Value of external version in breech presentation at term. *Med Tijdscher Geneested* 134: 2245–8

299. Van Dorsten, J.P., Schofrin, B.S. and Wallace, R.L. (1981) Randomized controlled trial of external cephalic version with tocolysis in late pregnancy. *American Journal of Obstetrics and Gynecology* 141: 417–24

300. Van Loon, A.J., Mantingh, A., Serlier, E.K., Kroon, G., Mooyaart, E.L. and Huisjes, H.J. (1997) Randomised controlled trial of magnetic resonance pelvimetry in breech presentation at term. *Lancet* 350: 1799–804

300a. Van Roosmalen, J. and Rosendaal, F. (2002) There is still room for disagreement about vaginal delivery of breech infants at term. *British Journal of Obstetrics and Gynaecology* 109: 967–9

301. Van Veelen, A.J., Van Cappellen, A.W., Flu, P.K., Straub, M.J.P.F. and Wallenberg, H.C.S. (1989) Effect of external cephalic version in late pregnancy on presentation at delivery; a randomized controlled trial. *British Journal of Obstetrics and Gynaecology* 96: 916–21

301a. Varma, R. and Horwell, D. (2002) External cephalic version should be routine clinical practice in UK. *British Medical Journal* 324 (7328): 49

302. Varner, W.D. (1962) Management of labour in the primigravida with breech presentation. *American Journal of Obstetrics and Gynecology* 84: 876–83

303. Vartan, C.K. (1940) Cause of breech presentation. *Lancet* 1: 595

304. Vause, S., Hornbuckle, J. and Thornton, J.G. (1997) Palpation or ultrasound for detecting breech babies. *British Journal of Midwifery* 6: 318–19

305. Viegas, O.A.C., Arulkumaran, S., Gibb, D.M.S. and Rathan, S.S. (1984) Nipple stimulation in late pregnancy causing fetal brachycardia. *British Journal of Obstetrics and Gynaecology* 91: 364–6

306. Wagner, M. (1994) *Pursuing the Birth Machine: The Search for Appropriate Birth Technology*. Ace Graphics, Sydney

307. Wagner, M. (2000) Choosing a caesarean section. *Lancet* 356: 1677–80

308. Walkinshaw, S.A. (1997) Pelvimetry and breech delivery at term. *Lancet* 350: 1791

309. Warke, H.S., Saragoi, R.M. and Sanjanwalla, S.M. (1999) Should a preterm breech go for vaginal delivery or caesarean section? *Journal of Postgraduate Medicine* 45(1): 1–4

310. Watson, W.J. and Benson, W.L. (1984) Vaginal delivery for the selected frank breech infant at term. *Obstetrics and Gynaecology* 64: 638

311. Weiner, C.P. (1992) Vaginal breech delivery in the 1990s. *Clinical Obstetrics and Gynaecology* 35(3): 559–69

312. Weissman, A. and Hagay, Z.J. (1995) Management of breech presentation: the 1993 Israeli census. *European Journal of Obstetrics, Gynaecology and Reproductive Biology* 60(1): 21–8

313. Wesson, Nicola (2000) Personal communication

314. Westgren, M., Edvall, H., Nordstrom, L., Svalenius, E. and Ranstam, J. (1985) Spontaneous cephalic version of breech presentation in the last trimester. *British Journal of Obstetrics and Gynaecology* 92: 19–22

315. Westgren, L.M. and Ingemarsson, I. (1988) Breech delivery and mental handicap. *Ballieres Clinical Obstetrics and Gynaecology* 2(1): 187–94

316. Wilcox, H. and Mo, B. (1949) The attitude of the fetus in breech presentation. *American Journal of Obstetrics and Gynecology* 58: 478–87

317. Wolf, H., Schaap, A.H., Bruinse, H.W., Smolders de Haas, H., Ertbruggen, I. and Treffers, P.E. (1999) Vaginal delivery compared with caesarean section in early preterm breech delivery: a comparison of long term outcome. *British Journal of Obstetrics and Gynaecology* 106(5): 486–91

318. Wolf, N. (2001) *Misconceptions*. Chatto and Windus, London

319. Wright, A.R., English, P.T., Cameron, H.M., et al. (1992) MR pelvimetry: a practical alternative. *Acta Radiologica* 33: 582

320. Wright, R. (1959) Reduction of perinatal mortality and morbidity in breech delivery through routine use of caesarean section. *Obstetrics and Gynaecology* 14(6): 758–63

321. <www.gentlebirth.org/archives/breech> Prenatal breech issues (30 May 1999).

321a. <www.caesarean.org.uk>

322. Zhang, J., Bowes, W.A. Jr and Fortney, J.A. (1993) Efficacy of external cephalic version: a review. *Obstetrics and Gynaecology* 82: 306–12

323. Ziadeh, S., Abu-Heija, A.T., El-Sunna, E., El-Jallad, M.F., Shatnawi, A. and Obeidat, A. (1997) Preterm singleton breech in North Jordan: vaginal versus abdominal delivery. *Gynaecological and Obstetric Investigations* 44(3): 169–72

324. Zlatnik, F. (1993) The Iowa premature breech trial. *American Journal of Perinatology* 10: 60

Index

Compiled by Judith Lavender

NOTE: Page numbers in *italic type* refer to figures and photographs.